One Tough Journey

by Bruce E. Jacobs

Edited by Jan Fitzhugh House

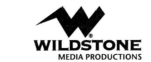

WILDSTONE
MEDIA PRODUCTIONS

PO Box 270238 • St. Louis, Missouri 63127
www.wildstonemedia.com

The opinions expressed in this book are solely the opinions of the author and
do not represent the opinions or thoughts of LCJ Enterprises, LLC or the publisher.

One Tough Journey

All rights reserved
Copyright © 2008 LCJ Enterprises LLC

Section III, Summary of Principles, and pages 70 through 92
may be reproduced for individual use.

Wildstone Media
www.wildstonemedia.com

First Edition 2009
ISBN-978-188246747-1

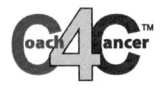

Coach4Cancer™ and C4C™ are trademarks of LCJ Enterprises LLC.

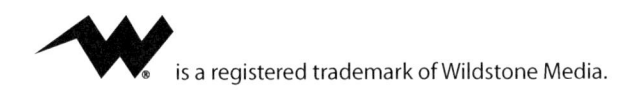

is a registered trademark of Wildstone Media.

Printed in the United States of America

Dedication

One Tough Journey is dedicated to newly diagnosed cancer patients and their caregivers as they begin *their* journeys through the cancer treatment and recovery process.

Purpose of this Book

As a newly diagnosed cancer patient, you now have a new purpose—to do everything possible to increase your odds of survival. The purpose of *One Tough Journey* is to coach you and your caregiver through the cancer treatment and recovery process. Cancer is not a destination, but cancer treatment is a journey. It demands you take a proactive role to help your body endure the grueling, toxic abuse treatment will inflict and to regain your personal power that many times will feel stripped away by the treatment process and the fear factor.

One Tough Journey shares what worked for me.

It describes my journey and the actions I took—from the first symptoms something was wrong to my diagnosis, treatment, surgery, a second treatment regimen and recovery. It also contains 15 easy-to-use charts, forms and journal templates that I developed after struggling through the same journey you are now beginning. Use them to help you and your caregiver become proactive participants during treatment and recovery.

I hope this book serves as a road map to guide your journey, help you endure treatment, subdue your fear and help you regain your personal power.

Table of Contents

Introduction

I was diagnosed with esophageal cancer in 2004. Like most newly diagnosed cancer patients, I entrusted my treatment program and surgical decisions to my physicians. They answered my questions during our brief appointments, yet, I felt I just didn't know enough to ask the appropriate questions. I was frustrated because *I didn't know what I didn't know*.

I researched the survival statistics for esophageal cancer, and learned they were about 15 percent. I knew if I was going to increase those odds, I had to become as knowledgeable as I could about the type of cancer I had, the prescribed treatment protocols, treatment options, recommended surgery and the physicians who would help me. I had to become a proactive participant and ask the appropriate questions.

With such a low survival rate, I didn't have anything to lose and knew I wouldn't like the alternative if I didn't do everything I could to beat the cancer. There was no silver bullet to make any of this go away. It was going to be a journey—*one tough journey*.

For me, the most unsettling aspect of the cancer treatment journey was I couldn't find a detailed, comprehensive source of information about what it would entail or how I should prepare and care for myself.

I didn't know if or *how* treatment would affect my everyday routines: Could I continue to exercise and work out? How much sleep should I get? Could I keep taking vitamins and supplements? What should I eat during treatment? Could I drink alcohol? How could I keep from catching a cold or virus?

As treatment moved forward, new questions arose: Could I prevent the diarrhea and constipation the chemotherapy caused? Was there relief for the neuropathy, the pain or the nausea? Could I keep from feeling constantly cold or stop my eyes from tearing? Which foods provided the highest nutritional value and cell rebuilding and recovery capabilities? Which foods contained essential antioxidants? What should I eat to improve my hemoglobin and red and white blood cell counts?

Questions are the heart of proactivity and cancer treatment participation. If you don't ask questions, the answers and information you need may not be provided voluntarily by members of your medical team. During an office visit, you have about seven minutes with your oncologist. That's not much time, and it may make you feel like you're on your own, without control or choices. But learning what questions to ask helps reclaim your personal power and gives you a sense of control over your destination.

My wife, Linda, was with me when my journey began and took charge as my primary caregiver during treatment, surgery and recovery. She did most of our research about the cancer, the treatment regimens, surgeons, hospitals, cancer centers, chemotherapy types, side effects, helpful antioxidant-rich foods, vitamins and many other issues we encountered along the way.

Linda gathered data and information, identified alternatives and options, worked with me to decide what to do and made me do it when she had to. She managed the process, administered the health insurance maze and told me when and where I needed to be for treatment, tests, blood work and doctor appointments. Linda did the real work. All I had to do was execute her plan. Linda's dedication and partnering were also instrumental in writing *One Tough Journey*, a coaching tool we hope will help newly diagnosed cancer patients and their caregivers prepare for and endure treatment.

For simplicity, the book is divided into three primary sections: **Section I** describes my journey—from diagnosis and treatment to recovery—and introduces the fear factor, its overwhelming presence and why you must learn to manage it.

Section II offers point-by-point information about what to expect from treatment and recovery and describes the principles and concepts that helped me survive treatment and its side effects. We separated these principles and concepts into three **"Must Get Rights":** Join the Journey, Feed the System and Decide to Live.

Must Get Rights

For easy access and reference, **Section III,** which starts on page 70, summarizes the **Must Get Rights,** and includes charts, forms and journal templates I designed for your use. These are perforated for easy removal so you can make copies. It also lists the online cancer resources I visited for information, support and reference.

One Tough Journey may not answer all your questions, but it may help you find them. The journey is tough, but not impossible. I have survived cancer to date and hope this book will help you on your cancer treatment and recovery journey.

One Tough Journey's 10 Primary Messages:

1. Decide to live—don't let your cancer's survival statistics rattle you.

2. Trust your oncology team to beat the cancer offensively with treatment.

3. Don't be afraid to challenge or question your physicians. They want you to win.

4. Be proactive and participate in your cancer treatment. It's your cancer.

5. Live through treatment defensively—with proper nutrition, rest, exercise and humor.

6. Feed the system—nutritionally, physically and mentally.

7. Get an attitude. Own your cancer—destroy it.

8. Find what works for you and never stop finding what works for you.

9. Consider your caregiver, for whom the journey is equally grueling.

10. You now have a new purpose. Go after it with a vengeance.

Section I:
The Journey Begins

*This section describes the cancer diagnosis,
the treatment regimen and how to manage
the fear factor that accompanies them.*

Section I: The Journey Begins

Getting the news you have cancer

There is no good way to be told you have cancer. Now that your worst fears and nightmares are real, what do you do? A cancer diagnosis is not a destination, but the rigors of treatment and its grueling, toxic side effects are *one tough journey*. There is no magic pill to make this journey go away.

Before you can settle your emotions around the fact you have cancer, your oncologist will have ordered a series of tests to calibrate your cancer and determine its stage and grade. Soon after, a treatment regimen will be prescribed, scheduled and started. Time is critical. Before you know it, your cancer treatment journey has begun.

My journey began Tuesday, May 25, 2004. Linda and I learned I had esophageal cancer just four days before our youngest son, Luke, was to be married. We were getting ready for the busy weekend ahead and looking forward to celebrating with family and friends—then

SLAM! I was ambushed by esophageal cancer. With the wedding four days away, my first reaction was this is not a good time to be diagnosed with cancer—but there is never a good time.

When I was diagnosed, I'd been married almost 31 years (to the same woman) and was the father of three grown sons: Robert, Nicholas and Luke. I had a successful career, and, though I'd spent sixty to seventy percent of it traveling, I'd always been healthy, physically fit and active, my weight always on the lean side.

However, I had smoked cigars for 25 years, finally quitting in July 2000, and I also suffered from some of the typical medical conditions found in Type A personalities with high-stress careers—high blood pressure, high cholesterol and acid indigestion—though all under control with medication.

Yet, the more I thought about it, the more I began to realize my cancer didn't just arrive overnight; it had been developing since early childhood, when I often suffered bouts of heartburn and acid indigestion. As I built my career, my colleagues and I used to say you knew who the best in our field were by the number of heartburn medicines they kept at their desks, and mine was no exception. With a professional career that spanned more than 28 years, I had worked side by side with many business owners and executives to improve the operating performance of their companies.

I'd recently changed jobs and had been with my current employer for only four months. Before I could build any momentum in my new position, I was ambushed by esophageal cancer. The toughest battle of my life and for my life had begun.

The first sign something was wrong with my body came one night in April 2004 while I ate dinner at a favorite restaurant with two of my sons. Linda was out of town, so the boys and I spent the day motorcycling and decided to ride over to the restaurant for dinner.

Our meals arrived and, as we began to eat, I started to feel extremely uncomfortable: The food felt like it was backing up in my throat and could not go into my stomach. I coughed, then gagged and had to walk outside to clear my throat. I returned to the table and continued to eat but it happened again. I went back outside, thinking the food may have simply gone down my windpipe.

When I returned to the table the second time I did not finish eating because I'd lost my appetite. I didn't think much of the episode, and the boys kidded me about whether I could ride my motorcycle home without tossing my dinner inside my helmet. I assured them that wouldn't happen and rode home without incident.

The following week it happened again—at a business lunch with several colleagues and at home during dinner. Linda cornered me and asked what was wrong. When I told her about the other incidents, she said, "You need to see a doctor." My annual physical was scheduled Friday, May 21; I would discuss the problem with my physician then.

In the meantime, I learned to manage any recurring episodes by anticipating the "clogging" and quickly clearing my throat. As long as I could keep adapting, I thought I could put off seeing a doctor until my physical.

After the exam, I told my doctor about the clogging in my throat. He asked how it felt. Where in my throat did I feel the clog and how had I cleared it? I said it felt like the base of my esophagus was blocked and food wouldn't drop into my stomach. He referred me to an endocrinologist who scheduled me for an upper and lower endoscopy on Tuesday, May 25—four days before Luke's wedding.

After the procedure, Linda and I waited for the results. Still groggy from the anesthesia, I was wheeled across the hall to a room with glass doors. Joking, I told Linda, "This is the bad news room where you wait for the bad news!" Sure enough, I was right—it *was* bad news.

The endocrinologist said he'd found a tumor: It was a condition known as Barrett's esophagus, the result of cellular changes in the lining of my esophagus. After many years of damage from acid indigestion, the tumor appeared cancerous. The lab would test a tissue sample to confirm his diagnosis, and he would call us with the results Thursday, May 27.

He was very polite, handed us a few 5x8 full-color glossy photos of the tumor and indicated the inflamed tissue he believed to be cancerous. I will never forget his next words: "This is a very serious cancer. You need to get your affairs in order."

With friends and family arriving from out of town, our home was in total chaos when the call came, confirming the tumor was cancerous. The doctor recommended an oncologist and would forward him the test results. When the call ended, Linda and I sat in silence. We were in shock. Our worst fear and nightmare were real. I broke the uncomfortable stillness and called the oncologist for an appointment; he could see us the next day.

Again the room fell silent. Finally, we started talking

about how we'd get through the weekend and the wedding. How and when would we inform family and friends? We decided not to share my diagnosis with anyone until after the wedding. We'd know more after meeting with the oncologist and could decide how to break the news then.

Linda and I had too much to do to just keep sitting there. We already had a full house with more guests on the way. Middle son Nicholas and oldest son Robert and wife Mimi had arrived from out of town, and my Uncle Ed had arrived earlier in the week. We were hosting the rehearsal dinner Friday evening in our home for more than 40 guests. The wedding was Saturday and Sunday we were hosting a brunch.

That afternoon Linda and I made three decisions: We would get through the weekend like nothing was wrong; we would share the news of my diagnosis after Sunday's brunch, before out-of-town friends and family returned home; we would not tell the newlyweds until they came home from their honeymoon.

I had taken vacation days that Thursday and Friday to prepare for the wedding and to enjoy some time with several of my bothers and sisters and their families. It was difficult not to tell anyone about my cancer. It was even more difficult for Linda to hold her emotions in check and not share the news with members of her family and our close friends.

Section I: The Journey Begins

Meeting the Oncologist

Friday, May 28—the day before Luke's wedding was "doctor day." Our appointment was at 2 p.m. We'd never visited an oncologist and didn't know what to expect. I'd been so busy getting ready for the wedding, I hadn't had time to form any expectations. I had buried my emotions and fears deep inside me to get through the wedding and the weekend. This weekend was not going to be about me. Whatever the oncologist had to say would not change anything about this special occasion.

My cancer treatment journey began with Dr. Alfred Greco at The Center for Cancer Care and Research in St. Louis, Missouri, which he and two associates founded in 2001. The center performs a blood analysis before every oncology appointment, administers chemotherapy in a large infusion room, takes x-rays, performs various scans, administers radiation treatment, fills patient prescriptions at an on-site pharmacy and offers many other services.

It's a bustling place, home to an energetic, cheerful, polite and helpful staff that's acquainted with many patients and their families. When we entered the main lobby, which also serves as the reception and waiting area, Linda and I were struck by the amount of activity. As center staff announced the names of patients, aids escorted them to have their vital signs taken. Other patients waited in line to report for their appointments, make insurance copayments or schedule their next appointments, tests and chemotherapy treatments.

We watched patients report their arrivals, pick up paperwork and head for treatment or to have blood work performed. Some placed paperwork in a box on the wall, then took a seat and waited to have their vital signs taken, while others waited to be called and escorted to an examination room.

Linda and I had arrived early to fill out forms, submit the insurance card, receive the admittance form and have my blood drawn for analysis. While we waited to see Dr. Greco, I became aware the patients seated around us were at different stages of the treatment journey. Several appeared very familiar with the routine I was about to learn. They were on a first-name basis with the staff, so I presumed they'd been in treatment a long time. There were other patients who, like me, were not well known; we were addressed more formally by our last names.

The number of men and women was about the same, and their ages seemed to range from the early 20s to mid80s. Many had lost their hair and wore hats, bandanas or scarves. Some were extremely pale, moved slowly and appeared somewhat feeble. Little did I know I would begin to look and behave just like them as I took my place in the treatment process.

Linda and I noticed most patients were with a companion—a friend, spouse, son or daughter, brother, sister or other relative. Patients did not talk to each other and seldom spoke to their companions. Despite the constant activity and cheerfulness of the staff, there was a serious sense of purpose and a strong awareness that cancer was no trivial matter. I sensed a quiet yet unmistakable anxiety, fear and nervousness in other patients; those waiting for their oncology appointments displayed a disquieting edge.

As we waited, we recognized that, while no one was happy to be there, some patients did seem happier than others. Whatever the type of cancer and whatever its stage, every patient and every companion in the waiting area were bound together by a common thread: hope—*hope* for good news, *hope* the cancer was in remission, *hope* that test results would indicate the cancer had not returned.

We met Dr. Greco who reviewed my medical file, the blood analysis results and photos of the tumor. He asked if I was in any pain and if I could eat and swallow. He thought I would require massive amounts of chemotherapy and recommended an infusion port be implanted close to the shoulder in my upper chest, which would allow easy access for drawing blood and infusing chemotherapy drugs.

Dr. Greco was very polite and appeared genuinely concerned as he described the severity and various stages of esophageal cancer and the types of treatment available. Before a treatment plan could be determined, I needed a series of tests to see how far the cancer had progressed. He answered the few questions we had, then told us it was urgent to schedule the tests—I needed to start chemotherapy right away.

We returned to the main lobby where we waited in line. One of the first things cancer treatment teaches you is how to wait, specifically, how to wait in line. You spend enormous amounts of time *waiting—waiting* to be called, *waiting* to have your vital signs taken, *waiting* for tests to be performed, *waiting* for the test results, *waiting* for the oncologist, *waiting* for the infusion nurse, *waiting* to be connected to the machine to start chemotherapy treatment and many other waiting-in-line events that occur throughout the journey.

Being really good at waiting in line is an acquired skill, one I hadn't mastered before I started treatment.

My journey gave me plenty of time to distill this skill down to its very essence. It helped me occupy my physical and mental energy during the treatment process, and it's a valuable skill I still use today when I have to wait in line.

My tests were scheduled for Tuesday, June 1, and port implant surgery would take place Friday, June 4. We also scheduled our next appointment with Dr. Greco, so he could explain the test results, the status of my cancer and the treatment he prescribed.

From the time we left the center that day to our next appointment, Linda and I hosted the rehearsal dinner in our home and celebrated the wedding. We also hosted the brunch for out-of-town family and friends returning home. As our guests prepared to leave, we quietly informed them of my cancer.

Earlier that day, so not to surprise them, we had shared the diagnosis privately with my Uncle Ed, our two older sons and daughter-in-law. Of course, everyone was shocked by the news, but we knew my cancer would disturb our sons the most. Their emotions ran high, from fear to anger, and they were bent on finding a cause to blame the cancer on. I made certain they understood I was not dying—I just had cancer and would tell them when I was dying.

Just as there's no good way to be told you have cancer, there's no easy way to tell your family, friends and colleagues you have cancer. You can sense the shock and fear when you tell people you're close to.

Even your closest friends can become nervous because they don't know how to respond.

There really isn't anything that can or needs to be said. Having been a cancer patient—and now a survivor—I've met and talked to many people at different stages of the treatment and recovery journey. I believe it's most comforting to simply say, "I am so sorry to hear this. I hope you do well with the treatment."

Section I: The Journey Begins

Treatment Begins

After the wedding, our guests returned home and Linda started her online search for information about esophageal cancer—the treatment protocols, survival rate, recent developments and the results of medical research trials.

Her research included general information about cancer treatment, chemotherapy drugs, treatment side-effects and the drugs that helped manage them, antioxidant-rich foods, vitamins, herbs, teas, nutritional products and anything else she could find about treatment and cancer cures. She also looked for information about cancer prevention and what would help the body endure chemotherapy and radiation treatment.

The week before my next oncology appointment, I had numerous tests, x-rays, scans and blood work. I drank CT suspension (which is like swallowing flavored Elmer's glue), was injected with test-specific dye and had the port implanted in an outpatient procedure at the hospital.

By now my concerns focused on survival. Though Linda's research hadn't confirmed the survival rate for esophageal cancer, we had an idea it was not very good. When we arrived at the center June 8 for our second appointment, Linda was armed with numerous questions for Dr. Greco.

We signed in with the receptionist and followed steps that would soon become an old, familiar habit: A copy was made of my insurance card, my appointment papers were handed to me, and I reported to where blood was drawn and analyzed. I returned to the waiting room, placed my paperwork in a box on the wall and waited to be called. Linda and I were new at this, but it was apparent we would repeat this protocol at every appointment for the next two years.

Like our first visit to the waiting room, we sat among other cancer patients and their companions. I sensed the same feelings of fear, anxiety, nervousness and edginess that I sensed during our first visit—only now I shared them. Soon we were called and escorted to an examination room to wait for Dr. Greco. He arrived a little hurried and disorganized but quickly settled himself and went to work reviewing my charts, test results and blood analysis. He asked if the infusion port had been implanted, then told us what the test results indicated about my cancer.

With confidence, he explained the treatment he prescribed, which had been developed and used successfully at the M. D. Anderson Cancer Center in Houston, Texas:

- **First round** – five days with Taxol, Cisplatin, 5FU; off treatment for three weeks
- **Second round** – five days with Taxol, Cisplatin, 5FU; off treatment for three weeks
- **Third round** – 25 days radiation treatment and continuous infusion chemotherapy of 5FU and Cisplatin; off treatment six to eight weeks for recovery

- **Surgery** – to remove tumor and majority of esophagus

The first treatment round would start Monday, June 14; the second round on Monday, July 12; the third round (radiation and chemotherapy) on Wednesday, August 4. Treatment would end Wednesday, September 8, with surgery scheduled for mid-October. Radiation treatments weren't performed on weekends or holidays. For them to coincide with chemotherapy, a nurse would disconnect my infusion pack every Saturday morning and reconnect it the following Monday.

Linda and I had many questions about treatment, its side effects, how to stay healthy and active and about my cancer's survival rate. I asked if I could continue to work out, lift weights and take my vitamins during treatment. Dr. Greco said vitamins wouldn't hurt me, and I could exercise but cautioned not to wear myself out.

Now that we knew the treatment regimen, I challenged Dr. Greco to be aggressive with it and either *cure me* or *kill me*.

In the days leading up to my first chemo session, I went through a full range of emotional and mental gyrations—disbelief, anger, self pity. My predicament and the low probability of survival had finally sunk in and hit hard as I wrestled with a profound awareness of my mortality.

Linda and I discussed our situation, the alternatives we thought we had and the choices we could and should make. Because my cancer's survival rate was so low, we agreed our best option was to do everything possible to increase my chances. I had nothing to lose, even if I lost the battle. I knew I could die but didn't think I would *lose*.

From Linda's research, we knew esophageal cancer was a very formidable enemy, relentless in its attack on the human body. At the time, I still didn't realize the toughest battle of my life and for my life had just begun. I *did* realize I'd made a conscious decision to join the journey and do all I could to survive.

The battle line had been drawn—the enemy on one side and my body on the other. Who would win the fight?

After cancer is diagnosed, your oncologist will prescribe a treatment plan and schedule. During our second appointment with Dr. Greco, Linda and I copied my treatment details on the back of a prescription pad. For your convenience, record your treatment plan and schedule on **Chart I**, *Cancer Diagnosis and Treatment Plan (p. 76)*, and **Chart II**, *Treatment Schedule (p. 77)*.

Before treatment begins, you'll also be asked to list your current prescription medications, vitamins, supplements and over-the-counter medicines. Record this information on **Chart III**, *Summary of Current Medications (p. 78)*, so it's available quickly on demand.

Section I: The Journey Begins

The Fear Factor

When you're told you have cancer, your mind begins to race with countless questions and concerns —all driven by fear:

➤ How bad is it?

➤ What is the survival rate?

➤ Am I going to die?

➤ What's treatment like—how long will it take?

➤ Is treatment painful—will it make me sick?

➤ Will I lose my hair?

➤ Will it kill me?

➤ Can I continue to work?

➤ Has it spread to other parts of my body?

➤ Do I need surgery?

➤ What are my options?

➤ Will my health insurance cover the treatment?

➤ Can I survive?

➤ Why is this happening to me?

The "fear factor" will consume you, and there is no simple means of clearing it from your mind. I had never experienced the level of fear I felt when I heard "It's cancer." I began to realize fear would be living with me for some time, accompanying me through treatment, surgery, a second treatment and recovery.

It was the fear of the unknown and what I didn't understand. Again, *I didn't know what I didn't know*. I had no idea what to expect or what would be expected of me—from the cancer treatment center, the treatment regimen, tests, treatment providers, surgeons, oncologists, my family and Linda.

As for my normal activities, I didn't know what I could and couldn't do as I went through treatment and recovery. Could I work, ride a motorcycle, play tennis with Linda, travel for work, lift weights, work in the yard, drink beer, take vitamins, waterski? The fear factor, and the questions I had about even the most inconsequential things, overwhelmed me.

When your cancer team describes the treatment regimen you're about to start, the fear factor begins to strip you of your inner strength and personal power. The unknown, not fully understanding what is happening to you, the belief you have few choices and little control—all these factors strengthen the fear factor's hold and this reduces your personal power.

You may begin to feel like a victim, and the barrage of tests can make you feel like a specimen. When you reach the point where you feel the treatment process is being done *to* you and not *with* you as a participant, it's the fear factor at work, pilfering your personal power. Don't let it happen. It happened to me and sucked away my energy, determination and sense of purpose.

The more Linda and I learned about every aspect of treatment and recovery, the more questions we asked and the more we learned. During appointments with your oncologist, you have roughly seven minutes of their time. It's not a social event; physicians are busy, but most will take time to answer your questions, explain the process and inform you of alternatives and choices. However, expect to take the lead and make the effort. It's about joining the journey and regaining your personal power.

You now have a life-or-death cause to rally for and participate in. Recognize your new purpose and do more than just show up for treatment. The more you learn about the process as a whole, the faster you'll regain your personal power. Join the journey and send the fear factor into remission.

Don't underestimate the influence fear can exert or its powerful physical and emotional hold. Fear can be come so excruciating during the journey that it sometimes causes you to act differently: You may get agitated and nervous, you may not sleep, and you may be unable to concentrate or think clearly. It can affect your behavior, temperament, health and the ability to make decisions.

Learning to manage the fear factor was essential for me because its intensity fluctuated. I still contend with my fear of cancer, and most cancer survivors will agree that learning to subdue the fear is the only way to live with it. The journey itself does not alleviate the fear factor, and even a long journey does not make it go away, yet there are steps you can take to alleviate your fear and regain your personal power.

> *The following worked for me and may help you*
> *subdue the fear factor and regain your personal power:*
>
> ➤ Develop a survivor's attitude to challenge a formidable, relentless enemy
>
> ➤ Decide you are NOT sick—you just have cancer
>
> ➤ Learn to manage the fear factor and realize you do have choices
>
> ➤ Make every effort to stay healthy during treatment and recovery
>
> ➤ Ask questions—don't be afraid to challenge your oncologist and cancer treatment team
>
> ➤ Avoid feeling like a victim by becoming a knowledgeable patient
>
> ➤ Join the journey—proactively participate in your treatment
>
> ➤ Believe you can win this fight

Section II:
Developing a Course of Action

This section defines principles and concepts designed to help you endure the treatment process and improve your odds of survival.

Section II: Developing a Course of Action

The Must Get Rights

Every cancer has a survival rate. When I discovered the survival rate for esophageal cancer was so low, I rationalized even a low survival rate meant *somebody* survived—why not me?

The research we accumulated about esophageal cancer—the treatment regimen, side effects, radiation, surgery and recovery—indicated this would be *one tough journey*. For me to survive, we had to learn how to improve my odds. It meant I needed to do more than just show up for treatment. It meant we had to develop a course of action and become proactive in the treatment process.

Linda's research also prepared us for the grueling abuse treatment would inflict: To kill the cancer, chemotherapy and radiation kill *all* the cells in your body, both cancerous and healthy. Clearly, the intent of treatment is to kill the cancer before it kills *you* or before it exhausts your immune system and must be halted before you get sick and die from something else, like pneumonia. We realized even the best cancer treatment would fail if my body couldn't survive it.

We were confident my medical team would do its best to play offense with the prescribed regimen. But treatment alone would not be enough. My challenge was to play defense and learn to help my body endure treatment and live through it. I'd have to get an attitude adjustment, stop whining and "buck up." I had to increase and maintain my body's strength. Surviving this type of cancer and its treatment regimen wouldn't be easy; otherwise, its survival rate would be higher. Over the next five months I endured chemotherapy, radiation *and* surgery. After my surgery in mid-October, I thought the journey was about to end—the chemo and radiation treatments were successful, and my surgeon, Dr. Alec Patterson at Washington University, found no evidence of residual carcinoma within the esophageal wall when he removed the cancerous portion.

However, in four of the five lymph nodes he removed, the pathology report indicated metastatic adenocarcinoma—in layman's terms, microscopic cancer cells. As a precaution, he recommended additional chemotherapy to destroy these cells, which he said wouldn't be visible on the numerous CT and PET scans that would be administered later.

After I recovered from surgery, my next appointment with Dr. Greco was Tuesday, November 23. He recommended I start chemotherapy again and prescribed the following treatment regimen:

➤ **First round**—three days Taxotere, Cisplatin, 5FU, Monday, Tuesday and Wednesday; the following two Mondays with Cisplatin and 5FU. Treatment would be administered over a three-week period, with no treatment the fourth week.

➤ **Five additional rounds**—same treatment as above, scheduled every four weeks

Before treatment could begin, a new set of scans and tests were performed to see if the cancer had spread to other parts of my body. The results showed it had not, but they didn't show any microscopic cancer cells either. Still, Dr. Greco and Dr. Patterson advised me to submit to a new regimen of chemotherapy to kill a cancer that didn't appear on the tests and could not be verified. It was a gamble: Was microscopic cancer still in my body or had it been removed during surgery? Should I sign up for the new treatment regimen? If I did, it meant starting the new year from an infusion chair, with treatment resuming Monday, January 3, 2005, and ending June 6.

At my next appointment with Dr. Greco, we reviewed the scans and tests results and discussed the proposed treatment schedule. He asked, "Are you still working out, taking your vitamins, drinking whey protein and doing the things you did when you went through the previous regimen of treatment?"

I told him I was and asked why he wanted to know. After all, I had questioned him six months earlier about continuing these activities during treatment, and he said *it wouldn't hurt*. Now he was saying, "Whatever you did worked for you. Your body adhered to the cancer treatment, and it worked for you." He even recommended an additional vitamin B complex to help protect my kidneys and liver.

His response forced me to reflect on the personal regimen Linda and I put together to help me endure treatment. Dr. Greco now credited it with my success. *Whatever I had done had worked for me…*

Was I missing something? Linda and I discussed what I'd done and what *she* had me do as my manager and caregiver. We thought back to the journey—to the events, tasks, research and actions we took. Then we distilled them into the principles called the **Must Get Rights** and grouped them into three categories:

➤ *Join the Journey*

➤ *Feed the System*

➤ *Decide to Live*

A brief overview of the **Must Get Rights** categories follows on pages 23 and 24; more detailed information about each one begins on pages 26, 40 and 58. As you review the **Must Get Rights,** you'll discover most of the cancer survivors you interact with have subscribed to many of its principles and concepts in one form or another.

You'll also discover proactive participants continually find *what works for them* and the difference this can make in any cancer patient's treatment outcome. To become a more proactive participant, refer to the "Find What Works for You" summary at the end of each category's section *(see pages 39, 57 and 67)*.

Before you begin treatment, prepare to devote every ounce of your energy to proactive participation in your treatment program. Be aggressive from the moment you are diagnosed. Get into an attack mode and begin the treatment process focused.

You may find the first treatment round is not too bad, but it will become more difficult as the fatigue

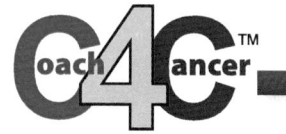

Must Get Rights

- Participate Proactively
- Be Knowledgeable
- Reduce the Fear Factor

- Eat Well for Strength
- Stay Active
- Develop Mental Fortitude

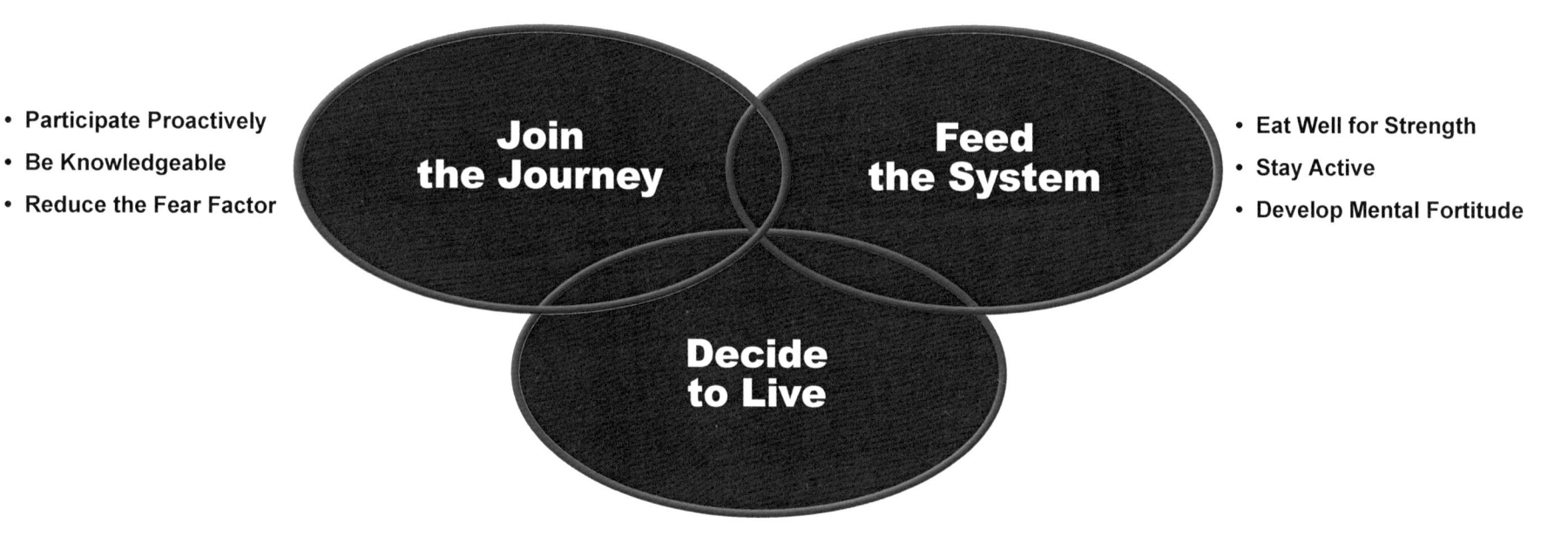

Join the Journey

Feed the System

Decide to Live

- Stay Engaged
- Buck up When Necessary
- Show Your Inner Strength

from previous treatments begins to wear you down.

For me, chemotherapy and radiation treatments were grueling, extremely tiring, and they also had a *compounding* effect. I later realized it was the little things I did on the treatment journey that became the core principles of the **Must Get Rights.** The following is a brief overview:

Join the Journey — The moment you join the journey you begin to participate. You begin to challenge your cancer and put it on notice you're in for the fight. That's when you begin to reclaim your personal power and subdue the fear factor.

The journey will become more difficult as treatment progresses and fatigue sets in. **Know this**: Every day will not be good, especially the days you receive bad news, but be positive—**you are not dying yet**.

Research your cancer and know your enemy. Learn as much as you can about treatment and its side effects. Engage your oncologist and treatment team and be prepared to ask questions and communicate with them. They will help you win this fight but you have to do your part. The more you know the more proactive you will become.

Feed the System — Cancer treatment engages your body in the worst physical battle it may ever endure. A weak soldier cannot survive a long physical battle. Stay strong during treatment and recovery: Feed the system the appropriate nutrition, as well as a balance of physical and mental activity.

This is the most difficult **Must Get Rights** principle because the treatment process works against you and your ability to feed the system. As treatment wears you down, fatigue sets in and you lose your appetite; you don't feel like doing anything and don't think clearly.

As the side effects set in, your fatigue makes them stronger, and it becomes even more difficult to be proactive and feed the system. This is when you must buck up and push through.

Decide to Live — When you where diagnosed with cancer, you didn't decide to *die*, but you probably didn't decide to *live* either. When you decide to live, you make a conscious decision to not just survive treatment but to live through it and become stronger because of it. Cancer is not a death sentence. You will know when you are dying and you're not dying yet.

You have to believe you will win this fight. Continue to live your life during treatment. Stay engaged with your work, social network, family and friends. There will be times when you feel you've had enough, can't take any more or go any further. This is when you must dig deep into your inner strength to meet the challenge, push through and decide to live.

Section II: Developing a Course of Action

Join the Journey

Many stories document the survival of cancer patients whose chances were very low. Most are ordinary people who were diagnosed with cancer and joined the journey. Not all are great specimens of athletic strength and physical fitness, nor are they wealthy celebrities or recognized authorities—just people whose lives were interrupted, or more realistically, *ambushed,* by cancer.

They joined the journey, dug deep into their inner strength and learned what worked for them to help them survive. I am a survivor—an ordinary, average person who was ambushed by a cancer with a very low survival rate. Linda and I knew I had nothing to lose, so we joined the journey at the beginning. Based on what I did to engage myself in the cancer treatment process, the Join the Journey principle consists of two concepts:

➤ *Proactive Participation*

➤ *Knowledgeable Patient*

The major points of these concepts are provided in summary form on page 27.

Proactive Participation

This concept puts your cancer on notice you're in for the fight, which increases your energy level and your commitment to survive.

- **Engage Your Oncologist and Treatment Team** — They want you to win your battle. Communicate with them to understand and assist in the treatment process:
- Ask questions
- Say how you feel physically and emotionally
- Tell them of changes and "events" in your body

It's important to have confidence in your oncologist and cancer treatment team. Don't be intimidated by doctors or staff. Change doctors if you're not treated with respect, don't feel confident about their capabilities or have difficulty communicating with them. **Chart IV**, *Questions to Ask in Treatment and Recovery (p. 79),* lists questions to use and build on to ask more.

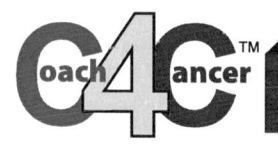
Must Get Rights

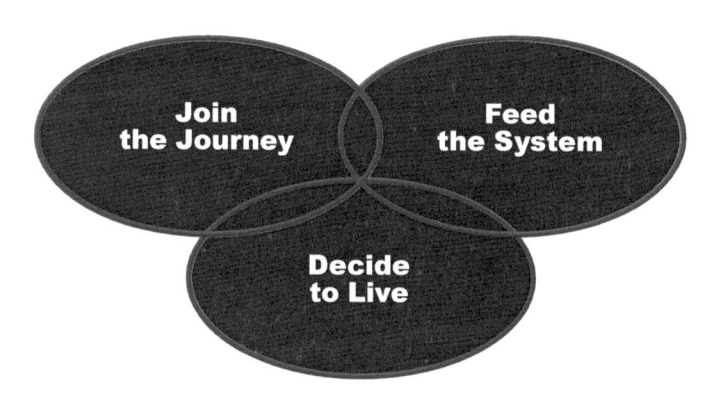

Challenge Your Cancer
Put it on Notice
You are in for the Fight

Join the Journey

Proactive Participation	Knowledgeable Patient
• Engage Your Oncologist and Cancer Treatment Team	• Research and Know Your Cancer Treatment and Its Side Effects
• Learn the Treatment Process	• Know Your Treatment and Test Alternatives
• Listen to Your Body	• Learn About Current Successes
• Prepare for Treatment	• Learn About Foods and Beverages Rich in Antioxidants
• Dress for Comfort and Warmth	• Recognize Your Temperament
• Make Notes and Prepare Questions	• Recognize the Toll on Your Caregiver

Find What Works for You

Linda and I asked questions that often began with why or what: Why are we doing this? Why is it a good thing to do? What does that mean? Why do you recommend that? What are you looking for? What does that tell you? Why is that important? The more questions we asked, the more we learned, and the more comfortable we became with the process. Before I started treatment, I challenged Dr. Greco: "Cure me or kill me and don't stop until I tell you to." In our ongoing appointments to evaluate my progress, his standard comment was, "I must be curing you because I haven't killed you."

Before every office visit, Linda and I talked about how I was feeling and about any aches and pains I had, then we each prepared our own lists of questions we wanted Dr. Greco to answer. At every appointment he would ask if we had any questions, so I'd pull our lists from my shirt pocket and we'd review them. During the course of treatment, the chemo created excruciating pain throughout my body. I felt like I'd been beaten with a baseball bat. The bottoms of my feet hurt, all my joints and major muscles hurt, and I couldn't sleep because of the pain. Linda informed Dr. Greco, who said it was from the Taxol chemotherapy and prescribed a strong pain medication I only took at night to help me sleep.

At another point, I felt unusually tired and my stamina was very low. When I discussed these physical changes with Dr. Greco, he believed there was fluid buildup on my lungs, ordered a scan to confirm it and prescribed medication to reduce the fluid.

- **Learn the Treatment Process** — Your medical team follows a treatment process; learn about it and ask questions. Understand what test results, blood analyses and vital signs represent and why each is important; be aware of any changes in them. These and other medical files are kept in your chart which is placed in a frame outside the exam room door. Don't be afraid to ask for and read your files while waiting to see your doctor.

Before you begin chemotherapy in the infusion room, an attending oncology nurse will take your vital signs and record them. It's a simple process with today's electronic equipment, so, instead of waiting for a nurse, I took my own vital signs—blood pressure, temperature, pulse rate and weight. I recorded the results on the treatment document I received at check-in. When the nurse arrived, I simply handed it over, proceeded to the infusion chair and waited to be connected to the infusion pump.

I found my chart and medical files very interesting to read, which helped pass the wait time. I was in the habit of removing them from the door as I went into the exam room. Before one appointment, my actions caused Dr. Greco to think he'd misplaced them, so he and the center's staff scoured around trying to find them. Then, a nurse watched me put them back and called off the search. If you're interested in reading your medical files, just ask a nurse for a copy.

The nurses will urge you to drink mass quantities of fluid to avoid dehydration, but the more you learn about the chemotherapy infusion process, you start to realize a high volume of fluid is pumped into your body along with the chemo drugs. You won't sit and relax in the infusion chair too long before you have to go to the bathroom, dragging the infusion pump and chemotherapy tree behind you. Try to come to treatment with an empty bladder.

Radiation is a trip unto itself. Before it can begin, technicians make a precise lead-based reverse mold of the area. In my case, front and rear molds were made from an x-ray type of scan of the area for radiation.

When you arrive for treatment, radiation technicians will select your mold, place it in the radiation machine and position you on the table for treatment. It's more like being fitted for a suit, only they put alignment marks directly on your body with a permanent marker.

I was told not to wash off the marks that were placed on my chest, stomach, right and left side and back. It looked like a basketball play had been written on me, but that's how the technicians align you perfectly with the machine that administers radiation. This process was very intriguing, generating what seemed like an endless list of why-and-what questions. By the time I started radiation treatment, I knew the process.

- **Listen to Your Body** — When you arrive for chemotherapy, you'll be asked how you're feeling. Describing how you currently feel and how you have felt since your last appointment or treatment provides valuable information for your oncologist and your team. **Chart V,** *Journal of Physical Health (p. 80),* will help you make notes, record how you feel and document any physical changes. Give your body the attention it deserves. Listen to what it tells you, especially as treatment continues and your side effects get stronger.

> *Your body will alert you to anything new or different. Pay close attention if you experience the following:*
> - ➤ Fatigue
> - ➤ Hunger
> - ➤ Pain
> - ➤ Cramps
> - ➤ Weakness
> - ➤ Dehydration
> - ➤ *Anything* new or unfamiliar

In treatment, my body went through cycles: It tolerated the first two days, but constipation set in the third and all hell broke loose by the sixth. Medication helped keep the nausea in check, but the steroids that accompany chemotherapy don't let you get a good night's sleep.

I was also very aware of my dry skin, joint and muscle pain and the numbness in my extremities. I was dehydrated, tired, fatigued and always cold. Yet, during the entire cancer treatment process and surgery, I never thought I would die because my body never told me it was dying. I knew I *could* die but I wasn't dying yet.

- **Prepare for Treatment** — Chemotherapy is a good thing, but it's also grueling, abusive and toxic. You may have to get psyched up for it because you'll feel exhausted at the end of each treatment session and will be even more exhausted the following day.

Get a good night's sleep before every treatment session. Be sure your body is operational before you arrive. Eat a good meal at least an hour before, attend to your basic bodily functions, bring your metabolism up to speed with a short walk and be ready to go.

Establish a mind-set that it's alright to wait in line and be patient. Plan how you'll use the time you spend in the infusion chair—write your notes and questions, document how you feel or outline the topics and issues you want to cover with your oncologist and cancer treatment team.

To develop questions and make notes about treatment and your body, use **Chart VI**, *Journal of Notes and Questions (p. 81)*. **Chart VII**, *Treatment Preparation Action Plan (p. 82)*, will help you get ready and plan how you'll use your time.

I used the time differently depending on the day of the week. Infusion chairs recline to an almost horizontal position so you can sleep; by Thursday or Friday I was so fatigued I did little else but. Generally, I caught up with my reading—the daily newspaper, business magazines and journals and other publications I subscribed to.

I worked on good days when I had the energy and always took my cell phone to make and take calls. My clients never knew I was receiving my daily dose of *bug killer* while we talked. When I was scheduled for treatment, I planned ahead to use the time effectively.

During my second session I wrote two articles for a client newsletter published by my firm.

- **Dress for Comfort and Warmth** — Wear clothing that provides easy access to your infusion port or other areas of your body where infusion will take place. Dress warmly in every season because chemotherapy drugs may make you feel cold.

I had chemotherapy in both the summer and winter; regardless of the season I always felt cold. I never felt this kind of chill until I started cancer treatment, so I always dressed warmly. The infusion room had blankets that were sometimes heated.

Since each of my treatment sessions lasted four to five hours, I often brought fruit, nuts and a thermos of green tea for my morning snack. I sometimes brought a high-protein meal substitute drink Linda would make with whole milk or half and half.

- **Make Notes, Prepare Questions** — After you're more familiar with the treatment process, newspaper articles and oncology magazines may inspire questions about cancer, treatment, new protocols and trials. You can never ask too many questions about treatment or your prescribed regimen.

Every cancer patient guide encourages questions, but how do you ask the right ones if you *don't know what you don't know*? Put your head into the process and write down whatever you're concerned about or ask a nurse, friend, caregiver or another cancer patient to help you develop questions.

The more questions you have answered, the more you'll know. This helps generate more questions about other treatment issues you experience. **There are no wrong or stupid questions about cancer. Chart VIII**, *Medical Appointment Agenda (p. 83 – 84)*, will help you prepare for your oncology appointments and prepare questions.

Document how your body reacts to treatment. Note sensory changes and how your memory and ability to think clearly are holding up. Document the following: nausea, diarrhea and constipation; changes in appetite, strength, stamina, breathing and sleep habits; hair loss, muscle and joint stiffness, stomach cramps, intestinal gas, body rashes, bruises, bumps, bleeding, thirst, dry skin—anything and *everything* that's different about you since you started treatment. Use **Chart IX**, *Journal of Treatment Side Effects (p. 85)*, to record this information, describe how you feel and to develop more questions and discussions with your oncologist. The more answers you have, the more you'll participate and reduce your fear factor. **If you believe you need a second opinion about a diagnosis or course of treatment, note and ask about it.** It's incumbent on you to request a second opinion or another point of view. **It's your life—take control.**

After I was connected to the infusion pump and chemo tree to receive my first round of treatment, the infusion nurse read an endless list of the potential chemotherapy drug side effects I could experience. By the time the nurse finished reading the list, I had already concluded *everything* that happened to me going forward would be a chemotherapy side effect. I became alert to any changes in my body that might be due to treatment and noted them. The more notes I made about my side effects—and anything else I could blame on the cancer treatment—the more I appreciated the *good days* I had.

As treatment continued, my side effects and pain became worse and I experienced "chemobrain." I don't know where the term originated, and it may not be a recognized side effect, but any cancer patient or infusion room nurse can tell you what it is.

Chemobrain mostly put my mind in a fog. My reaction times were very slow and my ability to concentrate was shot. It was difficult to read and comprehend for long periods and driving was mentally exhausting. The best I can describe it, chemobrain was like watching myself in a movie where the things I did and said and the way I behaved were different than normal, and I couldn't prevent or stop it.

One Saturday, my oldest son Robert called to check how treatment was going and how I was feeling. We talked awhile, then he asked to speak to his mother. Now, I knew Linda was upstairs, but I told him she had gone on a cruise with her family. He asked why she would do that, considering I was in treatment and would have surgery in about two weeks. I told him I was fine and that she would be back in two weeks, in time for the surgery.

Linda's family had actually scheduled a cruise, but she had cancelled because of my treatment and surgery. When our conversation ended, Robert immediately called Luke, his youngest brother who lived near us, and asked, "What is mom doing on a cruise with her family?" Laughing, Luke said, "What the hell are you talking about? Mom is not on a cruise; she's at home with dad. I just talked with her yesterday."

Later, I was told there were quite a few occasions during my treatment journey when colleagues, family members and even Linda thought chemobrain had prevailed.

Knowledgeable Patient

Cancer treatment is like playing high-stakes poker: the hope is that you are physically strong enough to endure the prescribed treatment regimen before becoming too weak, sick or toxic to continue it. This concept helps you become resourceful and allows you to contribute to the treatment process and your cancer team's efforts.

- **Research and Know Your Cancer, the Treatment Regimen and its Side Effects** — Know your cancer enemy. Learn the success rates of treatment regimens and trials. Learn about treatment alternatives and the survival rate for your cancer's stage and grade. Learn who the leading researchers are for your specific cancer and which cancer hospitals are treatment leaders. Visit the websites of the American Cancer Society, National Cancer Institute and the Wellness Community, all listed on **Chart XV**, *Resources (p. 92)*. Specific cancer centers and hospitals have online resources, and many websites address specific cancers — breast cancer, leukemia, lung cancer and others. If you don't have Internet access, most public libraries, and some churches, do.

  As you research your prescribed treatment, learn about its side effects and the potential damage it could do to other parts of your body, such as your kidneys, liver, heart and lungs. Learn how to combat the side effects and how to protect or strengthen other parts of your body that could be affected. Some side effects are known to vary in severity, depending on the patient and treatment dosage.

  Again, learn what to expect and be sure to note the side effects you experience on **Chart IX**, *Journal of Treatment Side Effects (p. 85)*.

- **Know Treatment and Test Alternatives** — For many cancer patients, this is their first experience with a serious, life-threatening medical condition. As you discuss treatment with your oncologist, ask what other treatment regimens have been recorded, what alternative treatments can be used and what their success rates are. Know your alternatives and their consequences. If you're not comfortable with a series of required tests and biopsies, question the need for them. You have a choice: If a procedure doesn't feel right, don't agree to it until it does. If the answers you get don't satisfy you, get a second opinion right away. Review your options but decide quickly because cancer doesn't stop—it works on you 24/7.

- **Learn About Current Successes** — As your research continues, look for documented success stories. Discern what these patients did to improve their survival rates. Talk to other cancer patients and survivors and learn what they are doing or what they did to survive. Every cancer survivor knows what worked for them, and I've yet to meet one who is unwilling to talk about their cancer, their treatment and their success.

  Look around—the best source of first-hand information may be sitting beside you in the waiting room or in the infusion chair next to yours.

- **Learn About Foods and Beverages Rich in Antioxidants** — Discover the foods, vitamins and beverages you should consume that are high in antioxidants and cancer-fighting capabilities. If you never paid much attention to antioxidants before you were diagnosed with cancer, the main sources are found in a large variety of fruits, vegetables, grains, green teas and certain other beverages. **Chart X**, *Antioxidant-rich Foods (p. 86)*, lists many of these foods and beverages.

- **Recognize Your Temperament** — It's extremely difficult *not* to be irritable when you feel like crap. The shock, fear, anger and emotional roller coaster that follow a cancer diagnosis can make you feel irritable, edgy and self-centered. Because your caregiver experiences your behavior, ask them about your temperament.

  They may not want to answer truthfully for fear of retribution—which also may indicate a change in your temperament. Your caregiver wants you to win and will do whatever it takes for you to succeed, so be careful not to bludgeon them and the others around you who are there to help. Don't expect anyone to know or understand what or how you feel, but if you drive your care giver away, you may not like the alternative.

My temperament fluctuated with how I felt physically. As cancer treatment wore me down during the week, I became edgy and irritable about *everything*. By my last treatment on Friday, Linda didn't want anything to do with me. A few days after I completed a week's round of treatment, I began to feel better and became less irritable.

- **Recognize the Toll on Your Caregiver** — Your caregiver's health and well being are of vital importance to you. Most cancer patients rely on at least one caregiver, yet the important role that individual plays is seldom if ever recognized in much of the available treatment literature. Because they are focused on treating the patient, even oncologists and cancer treatment teams seldom mention the caregiver's journey or take time to ask how they're holding up.

  Caregivers often suffer in silence as they prepare meals; transport patients to treatments, tests and appointments; fill prescriptions; wait in line; sit with patients during treatment; and perform many other activities patients aren't aware of.

Your caregiver had a life before you were ambushed by cancer, and it's important they not give it up completely. Recognize the toll your cancer has on them, including emotional stress, fear, change in lifestyle, little time for activities, fatigue and health concerns to mention only a few. Your cancer will disrupt your caregiver's life just as it has yours but in different ways.

My wake-up call came less than two weeks before my surgery. Linda's emotional stress and fear finally took their toll one Thursday. I came home from work and she said she wasn't feeling well—sort of achy with a headache—so she went to bed right after dinner. By Friday, the achiness had moved to her back and her headache was worse. We figured she had the flu and knew I had to stay as far away from her as possible; I slept in a different room, made my own meals and went to work. On Monday, things had not improved, and Linda went to her physician, who immediately admitted her to the hospital where she was diagnosed with meningitis. To determine if it was viral or bacterial, a spinal fluid sample was tested, but the results would not be known for three days.

Meanwhile, she was quarantined and given strong antibiotics in case it was bacterial. As it turned out, she had viral meningitis caused by high stress levels that weakened her immune system.

Cancer patients must be aware of how their caregivers are holding up against the stress and fear. If your caregiver goes down, you're in real trouble. Do whatever it takes to keep them healthy and encourage them to find ways of relieving the emotional stress. They may suffer in silence, but you don't want them falling on their swords.

Find What Works for You

Join the Journey is a commitment to participate in the cancer treatment process so it's done with you, not to you as a victim. What worked for me might not work for you, so find what does. This includes finding the right oncologist. A doctor who behaves in an aloof or cavalier manner, or is uncertain about the best treatment for your cancer, may make you uncomfortable. Should this be the case, change physicians, the sooner the better.

It's critical to have confidence in your oncologist and believe this is the person you want in the trench-fight with you. If you don't like the way your cancer team treats you, let it know how you feel. If things don't improve, change teams. You are not a hostage. If you think you need a second opinion about a treatment, test, surgery or anything concerning your cancer, then get one. If you don't speak up you may not like where you end up.

When I was diagnosed and Dr. Greco informed me of the treatment regimen, Linda felt I should get a second opinion. I said no simply because I liked Dr. Greco, had confidence in him and just wanted to get on with the process.

When it was time to select a surgeon, Linda and I again disagreed about getting a second opinion. I agreed to see Dr. Alec Patterson, another surgeon who had a very different surgical approach to removing the tumor and my esophagus. I'm glad I got a second opinion so I knew my alternatives.

Stay focused. You're in a battle for your life as the journey takes you through treatment and its regimens. Approach it with a passion and be intent on winning. What helped me stay focused was wearing a yellow Lance Armstrong Foundation Livestrong bracelet a partner gave me after I told him I had cancer.

The only time I've ever taken it off was when the surgical prep team had me remove it before surgery. I still wear the bracelet today because it reminds me of the journey and how far I've come since putting it on in June 2004. **It works for me.**

Section II: Developing a Course of Action

Feed the System

This is the most difficult **Must Get Rights** principle to get right. If you're starting chemo, radiation or a combination of the two, you must stay physically strong; yet, treatment creates a self-degradating cycle that couples loss of appetite and energy with many side effects.

Treatment makes you feel awful—you aren't hungry and don't do anything physical to create an appetite because you feel like crap, so you don't eat—a cycle that repeats itself in an endless loop. Sometimes it's a major undertaking to get up enough energy just to eat, and it becomes even worse because you lose your sense of taste.

As treatment zaps your energy, you may eat less and not feed the system properly, so your energy declines even more. During oncology appointments, your doctor will ask how you feel. You'll say you feel like crap, you ache all over, have no energy, no appetite and feel like a tennis ball is stuck in the middle of your chest that won't come up or go down (they call it nausea). The nurse who takes your vitals may say your weight has dropped and that you must eat or a feeding tube will be inserted.

This cycle is almost sadistic and must be actively broken to feed the system. Even the best cancer treatment won't succeed if your body can't endure it—beef up your system so it can. The actions I took to beef up mine became the **Feed the System** principle, which is defined by three concepts:

➤ *Nutritional*

➤ *Physical*

➤ *Mental*

The major points of these concepts are provided in summary form on page 41.

Nutritional Concept

Because cancer treatment reduces your immune system's strength, structure your nutritional requirements like an Olympic athlete in training. The foods you ate before your diagnosis may not be what you should eat during treatment and recovery. Modify your food and beverage consumption so it delivers the highest nutritional level to support your body's immune system, help you live through treatment and assist in recovery.

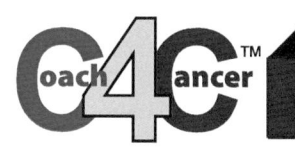
Must Get Rights

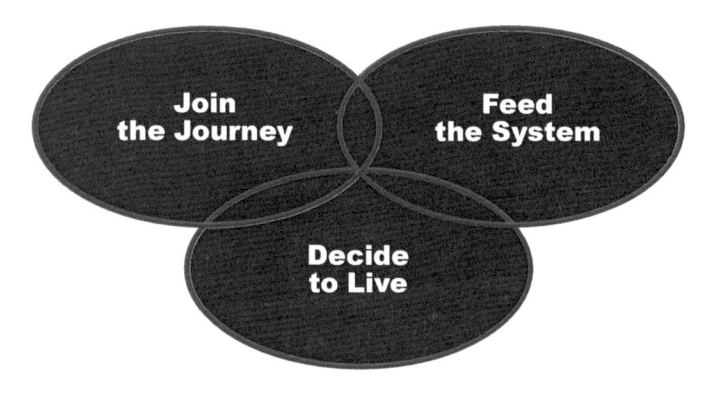

A Weak Soldier
Cannot Survive
a Long Physical Battle

Feed the System

Nutritional	Physical	Mental
• Eat Well for Treatment and Recovery	• Be Ready for Treatment	• Be Positive; Cancer Is not a Death Sentence
• Eat Four to Six Small Meals a Day	• Continue Your Normal Activities	• Dig Deep Into Your Inner Strength
• Eat More Protein	• Exercise and Play	
• Add Vitamins to Your Diet	• Sleep to Recover	• Embrace Your New Purpose
• Drink More Water	• Rest When Tired	
• Have an Alcoholic Beverage	• Work at Your Job	• Settle Your Emotions
	• Manage the Pain; It Will Pass	• Recognize Your Mortality
	• Document and Track Your Side Effects	• Stay Motivated
	• Nausea is Temporary	• Celebrate Small Triumphs
	• Hair Loss is Temporary	• Use Prayer for Strength
	• Stay Warm	• Plan Your Activities
	• Stay Healthy	

Find What Works for You

- **Eat Well for Treatment and Recovery** — To get the biggest benefit from treatment, feed the system nutritionally rich foods. Your body will weaken quickly if you don't eat balanced meals, including meat, vegetables, whole grains, fruits, nuts and foods high in cancer-fighting antioxidants.

  Missing a meal is not acceptable. Your energy level will rapidly fall, as will your ability to recover. Eat well before your treatment day begins and during it if your sessions exceed two hours. Certain foods and beverages will help reduce stomach cramps, diarrhea and constipation. Those containing folic acid (spinach, broccoli, lentils, citrus fruits, liver, fortified cereals and Vitamin B9) will help rebuild red blood cells.

Because my diet may have contributed to my having cancer, Linda revamped our meals and focused them around protein and antioxidant-rich foods like fruits, vegetables and nuts to strengthen my immune system and help fight the cancer. She devised a menu comprised of three primary meals and two to three smaller meals or snacks. We were concerned about nutrition and calories, not cholesterol. I wasn't overweight and have a fast metabolism, so losing weight would've been detrimental.

Green tea reduced my constipation, diarrhea and stomach cramps, and I ate a lot of berries, grapes and other fruits and vegetables, which also reduced the constipation. I consumed an enormous amount of nuts (cashews, pecans, almonds and peanuts), maybe because I could taste the salt. They were easy to eat and loaded with calories, antioxidants and protein. I dropped 13 pounds after surgery but gained back three before I started chemotherapy again.

I lost seven pounds during the second five-month chemotherapy session. I was pretty run down and my hemoglobin dropped so low I was almost anemic. It was essential to boost my red blood count and regain the body weight I'd lost, so Linda and I ate a lot of calf's liver, spinach, broccoli, cauliflower and grapefruit. There is a sample menu of those meals on page 43.

Sample Menu

During treatment, we rotated the following menus through the week to keep it interesting:

Breakfast: Several choices from protein-rich foods, along with cheese, fruit, a grain and beverage.

Protein — Eggs, Canadian or smoked bacon, prosciutto, smoked salmon, Gouda or cheddar cheese

Grains — Oatmeal or Cream of Wheat (with butter and half & half), slice of whole wheat toast, slice of cinnamon raisin bread or one English muffin with butter

Fruits — Applesauce, ½ grapefruit or one cup blackberries, blueberries, raspberries, strawberries, pineapple, cherries, cantaloupe, watermelon, grapes, kiwi, peaches or pears

Beverage — Hot green tea with honey

Midmorning Snack: One cup fruit, a banana, applesauce, pudding, 12oz. V8 or protein drink with half & half

Lunch: Sandwich of lean cuts of meat with cheese, olives, pickles, tomato, lettuce; cup of soup, fruit, vegetables or chips; iced green tea

Afternoon Snack: Two handfuls of nuts, can of sardines or oysters with crackers or 12 oz protein drink with half & half

Dinner: Several choices from protein-rich food, along with vegetables, grain, fruit and beverage

Protein — 4 oz serving of lean meat (chicken, pork, beef, lamb, liver or fish)

Grains — 1½ cups rice, barley, pasta, couscous or dressing

Vegetables — Red, white or sweet potatoes; 1 cup green beans, broccoli, spinach, corn, peas, Brussels sprouts, cabbage, carrots, zucchini, asparagus, acorn squash; or navy, lima or butter beans; mixed green salad with dressing; spinach with fruit, nuts and dressing

Fruit — see **Breakfast** list

Beverage — Hot green tea with honey, or ice water

Note: When anemia became a problem, I ate calve's liver at least once a week to help rebuild blood cells.

Evening Snack: Two handfuls of nuts, several cups popcorn or pretzels, can of sardines or oysters with crackers or 12oz protein drink with half and half

- **Eat Four to Six Small Meals a Day** — Your appetite will diminish, but you must continue to nourish the system. Frequent, smaller meals will make eating less of a burden, and you'll still consume the same calories you would from three large meals. Your primary nutrition can come from three main meals, with additional nutrition coming from two or three smaller meals or snacks. Eating every couple of hours will keep your metabolism up, stabilize your energy level and reduce the level of nausea you experience. **Chart XI**, *Meal Plan (p. 87)*, will help you plan your meals, snacks and other caloric intake during treatment.

I thought eating more meals each day would be a chore that would create interruptions. It took awhile to adjust to the smaller portion sizes, but they were easier to eat, and breakfast, lunch and dinner were still my primary meals. When treatment nauseated me, I found smaller meals went down easier and stayed down better.

Linda was like a military drill sergeant who was totally focused on the meals I ate and the nutrients I consumed. On more than one occasion, I pushed my dinner plate away after picking at the food. Linda would ask what was wrong. I'd say I wasn't hungry, I couldn't taste anything so I was finished. She would put the plate back in front of me and say, "If you can't taste it, eat it anyway. It's not about *enjoying* what you eat. You *have* to eat." I'd grumble, pick at my plate some more and would finally eat most of what she had prepared.

- **Eat More Protein** — Protein is a basic building block for cells and muscle tissue. Because the treatment process eliminates cells and damages tissue, eating more protein is imperative for growth and recovery. Many 12 ounce protein drinks are on the market that are low in calories and high in the vitamins and nutrients your body needs.

Most health and nutrition stores sell them: Ask to be directed to the protein products for weight lifters, and you'll find shelves full of whey protein products. The dry powder is the most economical and can be mixed with water, milk, half & half or fruit juice. You can add fruit and mix it in a blender. Also, there are protein drinks you don't have to mix—you just open the package and drink the product.

Nicholas, our middle son, is a weight lifter who has always used protein drinks to build muscle. Early in my treatment, he called to ask how I felt and if I was able to eat well. I said I didn't feel like eating but hadn't lost any weight. He suggested I start drinking whey protein as a meal replacement or supplement—it would be like drinking a milk shake.

At the time, *drinking* a meal was easier for me than eating one, especially if it was nutritional and added protein. I started drinking two protein shakes a day. The product was Isopure Whey Protein manufactured by Nature's Best (see **Chart XV**, *Resources, p. 92*). One shake contains 65 grams of protein, 210 calories, 3 grams of carbohydrates and very little sugar. I increased the calorie content by mixing it with half and half or whole milk, and my weight didn't drop during chemotherapy and radiation treatment.

Eventually, the chemo made me lactose intolerant, so I had to start mixing the whey protein powder

with water. It tasted terrible but, by then, everything did. Because I had to keep my protein level up, I later switched to an Isopure liquid drink that had 40 grams of protein and 160 calories. It resembled Kool-Aid but didn't contain any sugar. **Note**: The whey protein products I used were low in sugar and high in protein and nutritional value.

- **Add Vitamins to Your Diet** — Take vitamins during treatment to replace the nutrients your body loses as your appetite declines (see **Chart XIV**, *Vitamin List, p. 91*). Include the following supplements: a multivitamin, Vitamin A (people with cancer require higher-than-normal amounts of this antioxidant), Vitamin B-complex (aids liver function, helps build red blood cells and improves circulation), Vitamin E (a powerful antioxidant and cancer-fighting agent), Vitamin C (another powerful cancer-fighting agent that promotes the production of interferon in the body) and CoQ10 (improves cellular oxygenation).

Linda once had me taking so many vitamins they upset my stomach and made me vomit. With the nausea from chemotherapy, I could do without vitamin-induced nausea, so we reduced what I took to a multi-vitamin; Vitamins C, E, B; and CoQ10 supplements.

- **Drink More Water** — Drink as much water as you can. Treatment will dehydrate you if you don't consume enough fluid. Water is the preferred remedy to help with constipation and flush toxins.

I drank a lot of green tea. It tasted fine and was easy to make. It also reduced the nausea and the effects of diarrhea and constipation.

- **Have an Alcoholic Beverage** — If you drink alcohol, then have a drink to help you relax but be careful if you're taking prescription drugs; the alcohol could affect their potency or interact with them badly.

Linda once asked Dr. Greco if it was alright for me to drink beer while I went through treatment. I never asked this question because I didn't want to hear him say I couldn't. I thought if I don't ask, he won't say no. When Linda asked, I gripped the arms of my chair as I waited for the answer.

He told us it was fine but not to have more than two or three beers a day. Then he looked at Linda, and to my great delight said, "Beer is one of the few products cancer patients going through chemotherapy treatment can still taste." I said to myself, "Hurray for our side!"

In treatment I heard oncologists and treatment teams tell their patients they had to keep eating to keep up their strength and weight. Every time I heard this it sounded like a conspiracy—the treatment kills your appetite and makes you *not* want to eat anything, yet cancer patients are repeatedly told they *must keep eating*.

Again, it was the self-degradating cycle. The greatest proven weight-loss program in the world is chemotherapy. Anybody looking to drop 20 to 40 pounds should sit through a round or two and watch the weight come off. It might be expensive but it's effective. What better way to curtail your appetite or stop a bad munching habit? On chemotherapy, just the *smell* of fast food will make you toss your lunch and never set foot in a fast food restaurant again.

As difficult as it may be (and as often as you may be told to) you really MUST eat right and eat regularly while going through treatment. A weak soldier can't survive a long physical battle. Eat well to give your body every advantage. If you can't taste it, eat it anyway. It's not about fine dining. It's about *feeding the system* the proper nourishment to endure treatment, recover and survive.

Physical Concept

As treatment side effects set in, this concept will be more difficult to practice, but it may be what helps you stay the course.

- **Be Ready for Treatment** — When you're scheduled for treatment, be ready, get motivated and psyched-up. You can't expect a 100 percent cure if you don't participate. Eat a good meal, go for a walk or exercise before treatment and mentally prepare for it.

Before I left for treatment, my routine was to get up early, walk about a mile with our border collie, MacLeod, eat a solid breakfast and work out in the weight room for an hour. My body was operational when I arrived at the cancer center at 8:00 a.m. I was mentally and physically ready to be treated.

What started Monday morning as a commitment for a week of treatment always seemed more like a good intention by Friday. As the week progressed I felt my energy level decline. I'd walk a little slower each day, and my workouts became less strenuous. I could keep up the pace with MacLeod and do a full workout on Monday, but, by Friday, MacLeod was pulling me around the neighborhood, and my workout consisted more of stretching and lifting light weights. Not only did I lack the energy, I didn't have the strength (even with the steroids from the treatment) but I continued the routine because it kept me motivated.

- **Continue Your Normal Activities** — Just because you have cancer doesn't mean you can't continue your normal activities. As treatment progresses, your fatigue and lack of energy will reduce your desire to do just about *anything*. However, the more active you are, the less your mind will focus on the side effects and pain.

For me, staying active during treatment wasn't difficult but not having the stamina and strength I had before *was*. Linda and I remained socially active. I continued to work but curtailed business travel and cut my schedule to about six hours a day. My clients knew I was going through cancer treatment and were supportive.

During the weeks when each treatment lasted five hours, I went to the office for only three. At home, I continued to mow, trim, blow leaves and maintain the house, but physical work obviously took longer.

These activities didn't make the pain or side effects less tolerable but distracted me so I didn't dwell on them. Watching television was the most difficult because it didn't provide enough stimuli to keep me from noticing my side effects and pain.

- **Exercise and Play** — Get up and get moving. Go play. Ride a bike. Play golf, basketball, baseball or tennis. Work out at the gym, bowl, play cards, walk, swim, stretch or lift weights. Exercise and play will help you tolerate the pain and relieve the side effects.

Cancer treatment did not stop me but it did slow me down. I continued to lift weights but the workouts were not as long or strenuous. Linda and I took shorter motorcycle day trips with our friends. I still waterskied but not as long or as hard as before. On vacation, I even ran a one-week ski school for two of our nieces and taught them how to slalom ski, wake-board and knee-board. Exercise and play helped relieve the increasing side effects and pain or at least took my mind off them.

- **Sleep to Recover** — If you're not tired yet, you will be. Listen to your body and don't fight its need for rest. Steroids prescribed during treatment will disrupt your sleep pattern, so go to bed early or when you first notice you're tired. Sleep until you wake up on your own, which could be nine to 12 hours a night during treatment and recovery. Your body recharges, rebuilds and heals while you sleep; not getting enough reduces your motivation and energy level.

Getting enough sleep while in treatment was easy for me, though I didn't sleep during the day. I retired by 7:30 p.m. and woke 10 to 11 hours later. I always went to bed tired and awoke rested.

- **Rest When Tired** — If you're active, take care not to wear yourself out. If you work, take breaks and rest when tired. If you play, don't overexert yourself. You don't have to sleep—just stop and rest awhile.

Fatigue became a way of life when I went through the second five-month chemotherapy regimen. I don't nap very well and tend to wake up groggy and irritable, but I can catnap for 10 to 20 minutes without a problem. During my second treatment, catnaps rejuvenated me and didn't allow me to go into a deep sleep. I was cautious not to wear myself down. At work

or play, I did less and rested more frequently because I tired more easily.

- **Work at Your Job** — If you're employed and can continue to work, stay on the job if only part-time or on a limited basis. Working keeps you connected and involved and will take your mind off the cancer, the side effects and pain. By working, you send a message to yourself and coworkers that you won't let cancer strip you of your life. But pace yourself and recognize your limitations and reduced capabilities.

My employer allowed me to work at a reduced capacity. I could have gone on disability, and the firm could have asked me to, but it was gracious enough to trust my judgment about what I could handle. I generally wore out after six hours.

- **Manage the Pain…It Will Pass** — Treatment causes pain in various parts of your body, sometimes making your entire body hurt. Most of it can be managed with Tylenol. Excessive pain may require a stronger prescription pain reliever that, taken before the pain becomes severe, will help keep its cycles more tolerable.

The pain from chemotherapy was penetrating and all encompassing, from the bottoms of my feet to the top of my head. If I'd had any hair left I'm sure it would have hurt too. Though mostly tolerable with Tylenol, I ached so badly on one occasion that I couldn't sleep. I toughed it out as long as I could but finally requested a stronger prescription for relief. The pain was physically exhausting on the days it was really strong.

- **Document and Track Your Side Effects** — Treatment causes numerous side effects. It's not a matter of *will* you have side effects but *when* and how intense they will be. You may experience some or all of the effects the drug's manufacturer says are possible, including some not defined in the product literature. Every patient is different and experiences different side effects to varying degrees. When you start treatment, the infusion nurse will read aloud your chemo drug's known side effects. (Remember to note those you experience on **Chart IX**, *Journal of Treatment Side Effects, p. 85.*)

Treatment side effects were like holding a bag filled with unknown creatures: No one knew what I would experience or to what degree. The only known variable was that I would experience some or all of them. My side effects included nausea, pain, neuropathy, loss of taste, teary eyes, bleeding sinuses, dry skin, hair loss, loss of appetite, diarrhea, cramps, constipation, chemobrain, stiff joints, sore muscles, a sense of being cold and most of the other side effects commonly experienced. They got worse as treatment continued. Before every appointment with Dr. Greco, I documented my side effects and noted if they had become worse. For example, I first experienced neuropathy as a tingling and numbness in my fingers and toes. It became much stronger as treatment progressed and spread to my hands, wrists, forearms, feet and ankles.

- **Nausea is Temporary** — The nausea from chemotherapy subsides several days after you complete the treatment round. It affects your overall sense of well being and ruins your appetite. Eating frequent small meals helps reduce it. Eat foods that are easy on your stomach when nausea is strong and avoid those that are greasy, fried, spicy, sweet and hot.

For me, nausea was more of an annoyance that kept coming back like a bad dream. Green tea helped keep it in check along with the prescribed anti-nausea drugs I made certain I took during treatment rounds.

- **Hair Loss is Temporary** — Don't let hair loss disrupt your life or lower your self-esteem. It's a temporary major side effect from strong chemotherapy drugs, but your hair will grow back soon after you complete treatment. Use it to your advantage and, if you want, wear a wig, hat, bandana, or scarf. It does create a new look. Cancer patients know what it's like, accept it from each other and nobody else matters but *you*.

I lost all my hair during each major chemotherapy session. When it first started to fall out, I had it cut extremely short. I put on a bold and colorful print shirt, blue blazer, pair of khaki pants, a Yosemite Sam ball cap and my John Lennon sunglasses and went to the office. I told my colleagues it was my "Bruce Willis Country Club Look." Nothing more was said.

I eventually lost every hair on my body for a year. It started to grow back after surgery but disappeared soon after the second five-month session of treatment started. There are certain advantages: My bald head was easy to wash and dry, I didn't have to shave for weeks and saved money by not needing a haircut. When I finally did need a trim, I suggested my barber bill Dr. Greco for any lost haircut income.

- **Stay Warm** — Chemotherapy may cause you to feel cold more often. Stay warm, avoid getting chilled and cover yourself in treatment. The neuropathy side effects will make your toes, feet, ankles, fingers, hands, wrists and other parts of your body feel numb, so you may not notice when these parts of your body start to get cold. Protect your hands and feet from the cold in winter or they can suffer frostbite before you know it.

Cancer treatment changed my body's "heating system." The cold never used to affect me. I could tolerate the heat because my body would sweat, but treatment changed that, too. I *always* felt cold, which was a real nuisance during the winter because I could never get warm. My hands and feet were always cold and dry skin from treatment didn't help.

Even now, I must be very careful not to expose my fingers to cold temperatures or they will literally freeze. By the time they feel cold they've already turned white.

- **Stay Healthy** — Do everything possible to stay healthy and prevent infection. Avoid people who have a cold, flu or other virus. Your immune system weakens with treatment making you more susceptible to infection and other illnesses. Stay away from small children—they are germ factories. Wash your hands frequently and keep them away from your mouth, nose and eyes.

I was fortunate not to get sick while in treatment. The combination of eating correctly, taking vitamins, getting flu and pneumonia vaccinations and keeping my hands clean worked to keep me healthy.

Mental Concept

This concept is about having the right state of mind. It's about your outlook, attitude and motivation. It's difficult to have the right state of mind when you're in shock from the news you have cancer. It requires conscious effort to develop and maintain the right state of mind and a positive outlook and mental attitude— but keep working at it. Even with a good attitude you won't be positive all the time, especially if you keep getting bad news.

- **Be Positive…Cancer Isn't a Death Sentence** — Cancer is often curable. Survival statistics indicate more cancer patients survive cancer today than ever. **Why not you?** Once you're over the shock, take action. Do your part to increase your odds of survival and complement your treatment team's efforts. A 100 percent cure is only possible if you buck up.

This is a difficult high-stakes journey. There aren't many easy choices, but that doesn't mean it's hopeless. Focus your mind and prepare for *one tough journey*.

After I was diagnosed, it took me a few weeks to settle my mind and decide what to do. This wasn't a journey I would have chosen for myself, but I realized I had to take it on with the best of my abilities. I didn't want to tell myself later it was what I *should have done*. The more research Linda and I did, the more we learned and the more we believed survival was possible.

- **Dig Deep Into Your Inner Strength** — Draw on your inner strength and spirit during treatment. Both are powerful allies that can help you stay motivated and maintain a positive attitude. On occasion, your inner strength and spirit will be all that get you through the really bad days.

I had to dig really deep into my inner strength and spirit at least four times during treatment. The first

was when I became totally fatigued during my initial chemotherapy sessions and radiation treatments. The pain in my throat was terrible because radiation had burned the inside of my esophagus—I couldn't eat or swallow. In addition, the chemo made every bone, joint and muscle in my body ache with pain. I told a friend I didn't think I was going to make it through this, yet somehow I persevered and pushed through.

The second time was the day after surgery when I had to get up and walk with the physical therapist as I hauled my equipment monitor and IV pole with fluid bags behind me. After the walk, the therapist had me sit in a chair for an hour as part of my therapy. I never experienced the level of pain I felt while waiting for that hour to pass.

The third was after my surgery but before the second major chemo session: I had to dig deep to develop the willpower and motivation to go through it again.

The fourth time was during my second session, between the third and fourth round of chemotherapy. I was beginning to feel very run down and fatigued. The side effects were strong and the pain was equally high.

Dr. Greco asked if I could continue. I had to dig deep down to say, "Don't stop until I tell you to."

- **Embrace Your New Purpose** — If you ever needed a cause to rally around, surviving cancer is it. Focus all your effort on doing everything you can to improve your chances of survival. Your cancer will do everything it can to defeat you. Embrace your new purpose and work with your oncologist and cancer treatment team to defeat the cancer enemy. **Understand this:** You are engaged in a life-threatening battle with a relentless enemy determined to kill you.

Because esophageal cancer acts fast and has such a low survival rate, doing nothing *was* an alternative. But I've never walked away from a fight that was forced on me. As Linda and I talked about it, I figured this would be like fighting someone bigger than me—my opponent might beat me in the end but would get bloody doing it.

That's pretty much how I rationalized it and embraced my new purpose. It would be a good fight.

Even if I lost the battle, it wouldn't be because I didn't fight back.

- **Settle Your Emotions** — When you're diagnosed with cancer, your emotions rip through you like a roller coaster at a theme park. You may experience the emotional phases of disbelief, anger, self-pity and realization. The sooner you're able to process these emotions, the sooner you can focus your energy on the business at hand—survival.

During your journey, remnants of anger and self-pity may resurface—that's normal. These feelings aren't right or wrong but consume enormous energy so move on and don't dwell on them. For example, if you're worried about cancer recurring, worry after you complete treatment. Energy is precious; don't waste it. Reserve it and use it to endure treatment and help your body recover.

I was able to get through the emotional phases quickly and started learning how to improve my chances of survival; however, as my energy level declined and fatigue set in, it was easy to become angry about having cancer and indulge in self-pity. These feelings didn't persist for very long. After a good night's sleep, I reminded myself of everything I had: a new purpose, people who cared about me (and for me) and many things I wanted to do and complete.

- **Recognize Your Mortality** — A cancer diagnosis creates a powerful fear. It's especially unsettling if it's the first time you've reckoned with your mortality. Make peace with it. Once you do, your fear of dying will diminish.

Accepting my mortality was difficult. It took two months of cancer treatment before my fear of dying went away. I didn't want to die, but I knew survival would sometimes be out of my control during the journey. Trusting God helped me make peace with dying and helped remove thoughts of death from my mind. By the time I accepted my mortality, I was too preoccupied with chemotherapy, radiation and a host of side effects to waste more time wrestling with it.

- **Stay Motivated** — It's easier to *get* motivated than to *stay* motivated to undergo cancer treatment because it wears you down, dampens your spirit and reduces your determination. Be aware of this and talk about it with your caregiver, spouse, family or friends who can help you stay the course.

My motivation weakened when treatment took its worst toll—the side effects were intense, my energy and stamina low. Talking about how I felt with Linda and our sons helped me through these periods. My determination rebounded as I began to feel better.

- **Celebrate Small Triumphs** — There will be times you feel you've had enough. When it seems the journey will never end, it helps to acknowledge and celebrate every small triumph. You may not feel you're hitting any grand-slam home runs, but you will have hit a lot of singles. Bundled together, the small triumphs add up so recognize them: Your blood count hasn't declined as quickly as it had.

You've been healthy during treatment; some side effects haven't been too severe. You ate some thing you could *taste* and it actually tasted GOOD!

As I became more fatigued, celebrating my small triumphs made me feel better: There's only one more day of treatment this week. I won't have chemo again for 21 days. I can taste beer and peanuts—hooray for our side! Small triumphs became very important to me.

- **Use Prayer for Strength** — If prayer works for you, then pray. Let it create inner peace and settle your fear factor. Use it to get in touch with yourself, to be with God or both. Use it to build your determination and mental state to endure treatment. Never underestimate its power to give you strength.

Prayer was a way for me to retreat from the reality of the cancer treatment journey. It was comforting and gave me strength to endure what I was going through.

- **Plan Your Activities** — Plan things to do and stay active. The more active you are the less you'll dwell on your cancer. Try new things or do familiar things differently. You have cancer—what do you have to loose?

The motorcycle trips I planned were much shorter than those I'd taken before cancer, but they kept me active. Conducting ski school for my nieces was a wild idea, also one I *planned*. Every weeknight I planned things I wanted to do, and every weekend I did them.

I also planned to design two tattoos for myself: The first incorporated the initials of my sons' names in Gothic lettering; the second was a Celtic cross. Surgery left so many scars on the front of me, I looked like I'd been hit by shrapnel. My new tattoos wouldn't be noticed, so I had them inscribed before my second chemotherapy session. Being active didn't make the cancer, side effects or pain go away but it kept my mind off them and generally helped me fall asleep—and sleep well.

Find What Works for You

Cancer treatment takes an immense toll on your mental and physical strength, immune system and body as a whole. Improve your ability to endure the treatment so it defeats the cancer, not you. The Feed the System challenge is to find what works for you from a combination of nutritional, physical and mental concepts that can beef-up your system. It demands you and your caregiver participate in the process at the highest possible level. The more involved you are, the sooner you'll find what works for you, including the foods you eat, the vitamins you take, your exercise routine, what you do to stay active and engaged and how much sleep you need, to mention a few. You may find what *doesn't* work more quickly than what does so work at it and don't get discouraged.

Linda and I found many things that worked for me or solved short-term problems. I couldn't swallow after radiation treatment, so we had to determine what I could eat, or I'd be fed through a feeding tube. Soft foods that didn't irritate my esophagus and were easy to ingest worked for me: ham, tuna and chicken salad; pasta, mashed potatoes and soft meats with gravy; soups; hot cereals; poached eggs; warm tea; canned fruit, applesauce and any soft food in a sauce.

When my blood count was low, we learned what foods and vitamins helped build red blood cells. When my side effects or pain increased, we added two cups of apple cider vinegar to a hot bath. Talking with good friends, my kids and Linda about how I felt greatly improved my focus and motivation. These remedies were inexpensive, did not compromise my immune system and *worked for me*.

Section II: Developing a Course of Action

Decide to Live

Cancer is not always a final destination. When you decide to live, you refuse to let the cancer take over or totally disrupt your life. How you decide to live with cancer is your choice and one that will help boost your personal power. Deciding to live is not the opposite of deciding to die. Rather, it's the converse of *not living*. Do more than just survive the treatment—live through it and become stronger for it.

The two concepts that defined my decision to live became the **Decide to Live** principle:

➤ *Stay Engaged*

➤ *Get an Attitude*

The major points of these concepts are provided in summary form on page 59.

Stay Engaged

Cancer complicates your life and slows you down but do not let it stop you. It's more difficult to live life *with* cancer, but it's better than not living. Don't let cancer strip you of living. You have a life—live it.

- **Buck Up** — Not every day is going to be good. There will be periods when you have more bad days than good days, but they will pass. Prepare to dig deep into your inner strength because the bad days will be more frequent as the treatment wears you down. Sometimes the intensity of the side effects can make an okay day become a really bad one.
- **Believe You Can Win the Fight** — Don't let survival statistics convince you the odds are against you or that you cannot win your fight with cancer. To win this fight you must first believe you can. If you don't, you may never be able to commit to survival.

I knew my fight with cancer was going to be tough. With less-than-favorable survival statistics, I knew it was a fight I could lose, yet I never felt I would. As treatment continued and my tests began to show improvement, my confidence increased.

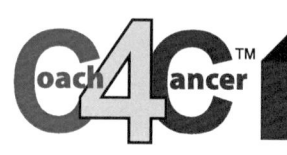
Must Get Rights

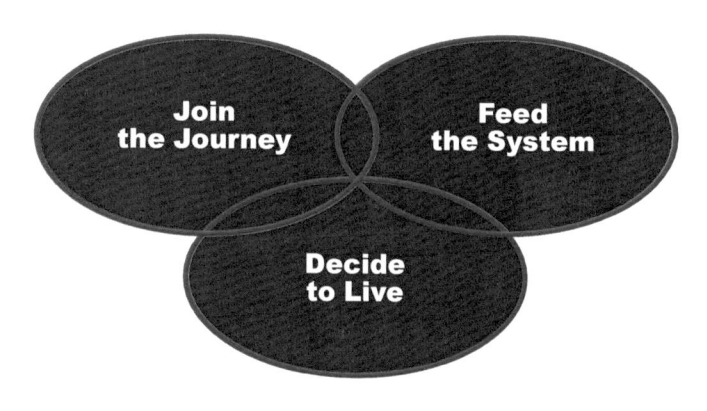

Challenge Your Cancer
Put it on Notice
You are in for the Fight

Decide to Live

Stay Engaged	Get an Attitude
• Buck Up	• Stay Connected with Your Social and Family Networks
• Believe You Can Win the Fight	• Challenge the Cancer
• Regain Your Personal Power	• Do New Things
• Continue with Your Life	• Choose Not to be a Victim
• Celebrate the Good Days and Push Through the Bad	• Don't Get Discouraged
	• Recover to Live
	• Call on Your Sense of Humor

Find What Works for You

- **Regain Your Personal Power** — Live your life and you'll feel less like a victim. Challenge the process and ask questions to help you participate and make decisions. Your oncologist, surgeon and treatment team will make treatment decisions for you, but as you regain your personal power, you'll participate in those decisions more often. The more you know about your alternatives, the more you'll be able to challenge medical recommendations and decisions. You may agree with your medical team but on *your* terms.

During my journey I challenged the process, the choices that were made for me and the recommendations I received. Knowing more about my options put me in a better position to decide what I wanted to do or have done to me.

For example, one discussion with Dr. Greco was about whether it was better for treatment to follow surgery or for surgery to follow treatment. After he explained my options and benefits, I agreed with his recommendation for aggressive treatment followed by surgery.

Another instance involved the choice of a surgeon and the best surgical approach. Linda and I asked Dr. Greco to recommend a surgeon, but we also did our own search and chose Dr. Patterson because we favored his surgical procedure and his experience.

Following surgery, I challenged the hospital's recommended recovery stay of 12 to 14 days and was released after only eight. While I recovered, I also asked Dr. Greco if it would be all right to inscribe the tattoos I had designed. He preferred I wait but I did it anyway.

I also had a choice about treating the microscopic cancer cells found in my lymph nodes: Should I wait to see if the cancer was still in my body and would return later, or should I start the second five-month session of chemotherapy? The data indicated no difference in the survival rates, but we decided to proceed with the treatment anyway.

The last major incident I'll describe was with an ophthalmologist. Chemotherapy had closed my tear ducts so my eyes teared constantly. To remedy this, he recommended surgically inserting glass tubes into my tear ducts to keep them open. My alternative? He could clear them with irrigation once a week and prescribe a steroid-based tear drop I could use to keep them open. I chose weekly irrigation and eye drops. Two weeks after my last treatment round, my eyes cleared on their own.

Like it or not, the treatment process is done to you. It can be overwhelming and frightening and can strip you of your personal power if you let it. Assert yourself and become part of the process. Regain your personal power, explore your options and reduce the fear factor.

- **Continue with Your Life** — You had a life before your cancer diagnosis and treatment and neither is a mandate to discontinue your life. **Keep living.** Do the things you did before to the extent you feel up to doing them. You will definitely feel less like doing a lot of things—even things you love to do. Just do them at a slower pace.

Do not become sedentary.

I tried to continue what I did before cancer—I just had a new companion along for the ride, and the treatment effects were extra baggage. Linda and I felt we still had a lot of living to do and decided not to let cancer waste our opportunity to keep living our lives.

- **Celebrate the Good Days and Push Through the Bad** — There may be times during treatment when there aren't any good days. Bad days rack up when treatment wears you down and fatigue sets in. When you have a good day make sure to enjoy it. Do something you've felt too poorly to do. Do something new and different. Celebrating the good days helps build your inner strength, adds to your personal power, strengthens your motivation and reinforces your belief you can get through this.

My problem celebrating good days was I would overdo it and pay the next day with increased fatigue. I needed to pace myself and expend less energy, so Linda and I began celebrating the good days by riding our motorcycles to the local bakery for a cinnamon roll or to a barbecue restaurant for lunch. Linda needed her "hit" of bakery sweets, and I could still taste smoked barbecue.

Get an Attitude

There is no reason to be humble in your fight against cancer. To defeat your enemy, get an attitude that puts your cancer on notice you are ready to fight and win. The attitude you develop will help you stay motivated.

- **Stay Connected with Your Social Networks** — Don't retreat or become a recluse. If you weren't a recluse before cancer, there is no reason to become one now. When you meet with family and friends, tell them you have cancer. Show your resolve that cancer isn't going to take over your life.

Linda and I both come from large families; between the two, you could spend every weekend at some kind of family event. We continued to participate in these activities and in those with friends. My personal attitude: "I'm not dying; I've just got cancer."

- **Challenge the Cancer** — Fight back and do not intend to lose. This is the attitude you need to subdue the fear factor and stay motivated. It allows you to draw on your inner strength when you need it most.

I fundamentally believed *everything* I did challenged my cancer. This gave me the inner strength to stay motivated and not give up. It was not about being *positive*—it was about commitment and determination not to let cancer win the fight.

- **Do New Things** — If there is something you've always wanted to do but have always put it off, why wait any longer? Do it! Live your life. It doesn't have to be expensive or elaborate. It can be anything—get that tattoo; dress differently;

eat new foods; go to the movies, a play, the ball game or go ice skating.

My new things included running a waterski school for two of our nieces, riding my motorcycle to church on Sundays, designing two new tattoos and having them inscribed and spending more time with my family.

- **Choose Not to be a Victim** — This is a choice only you can make. Cancer treatment will make you feel like a victim at some point on the journey but don't become a victim by default. Stay engaged, become *proactive* and *participate*.

I felt like a victim when I couldn't control what was happening to me. Having surgery and recovering in the hospital made me feel like a victim. I knew I wasn't a *customer* so I must have been a victim. I even felt like a specimen on several occasions.

Maybe the medical system is designed to make patients feel like victims and specimens, so they get healthy and *stay* healthy. If patients were treated like customers, they would keep coming back.

- **Don't Get Discouraged** — It's easy to get discouraged because treatment can lower your determination and your inner strength to continue the battle. It's very difficult to be positive when the news is not good, but it's not about being positive—it's about maintaining your confidence and believing you can beat cancer.

- **Recover To Live** — When you complete treatment, the cancer journey isn't over yet. It moves into recovery, a new phase where you rebuild and strengthen your blood count, stamina, energy and immune system. The "soldier" is tired and needs rejuvenation. Your appetite will return, the nausea will disappear, and many of the side effects will decrease or go away. Appropriate nutrition is essential to rejuvenate your body and help it recover. As in treatment, develop a meal plan. Select foods, vitamins, meal supplements, whey protein drinks, herbs and other products that provide the highest nutritional value. Eat foods that raise your blood hemoglobin level; as it improves so will your stamina.

Increase your physical activity and exercise to build strength and stamina. Regular exercise also helps relieve neuropathy and numbness in your hands and feet. As your body regains strength, your ability to concentrate will return. Focus on becoming as strong and healthy as possible for two reasons: **to prevent the cancer from returning and to be strong enough to endure treatment if it does.**

Don't expect a "Certificate of Completion" when you finish your final treatment round. You'll say goodbye to the staff at your treatment facility and walk out the door. You'll only return for follow-up appointments with your oncologist.

Before you start recovery, develop a recovery plan and discuss it with your oncologist.

Depending on the treatment level you endured and how exhausted you are, it could take 12 to 24 months to recover your strength, stamina and former body weight. A recovery plan and journal are essential. **Chart XII**, *Recovery Plan and Journal (p. 88 – 89)*, and **Chart XIII**, *Recovery Schedule (p. 90)*, are provided to help you.

- **Call on Your Sense of Humor** — Laughter has a medicinal effect. Let your sense of humor ease the treatment torment of the long journey and subdue the fear factor. Cancer centers, infusion areas, radiation and test rooms may not seem conducive to humor, but in certain situations, the treatment process is ripe for laughter.

My sense of humor has always created trouble for me and this journey was no exception. I agree cancer is not a humorous subject. It's difficult to joke about sitting in an infusion chair while chemotherapy tries to kill every cell in your body along with the cancer. But, *it is what it is*—finding the humor in it makes it more tolerable and alleviates the fear.

Somehow I've always found the humor in most situations, and the treatment process is an ideal setting because humor is so unexpected. I also use humor as a defense mechanism to help me endure life's frustrations; during the treatment journey I found numerous occasions for levity.

Following is a list I developed of the *good* things about cancer treatment and a list of humorous responses I used when answering questions my medical team asked during the treatment process. Add yours to either list—there's more humor out there.

Good Things About Cancer Treatment:

- Mosquitoes and chiggers won't bite you.
- You can get steroids legally.
- It's a great weight-reduction program.
- You might qualify for handicapped parking.
- You don't have to shave—anywhere.
- A bald head is easy to dry after a shower.

Responses:

- I felt OK when I got here.
- I'm retaining fluids?
  Hell, I'm glad I can retain anything.
- My barber's billing my oncologist for lost haircut revenue.
- Do I get a "Certificate of Suffering" for finishing treatment?
- Does treatment come with a warranty?

My last chemo treatment was June 6, 2005. I felt a little better each day that followed, but it took 18 months before I felt really good again. I still have neuropathy and my sense of taste has not returned, but I feel pretty strong and healthy. My stamina is good and my appetite continues to improve.

When I completed my last treatment I thought it strange to simply get up and walk away. I spent the better part of a year in that treatment room—five days a month with numerous blood tests every month and sometimes twice a month. Now it was over. It felt like driving out of a small town: I stopped at the last light and waited for it to change before rolling out of town and down the road on my new journey—cancer *survivor*.

There was no Certificate of Completion, no Award for Endurance, no congratulations for surviving and completing the treatment regimen. There were no good-byes or good-lucks from the treatment room staff as I waved and walked out the door.

When Linda and I arrived for the next appointment, we asked Dr. Greco what we should do to improve my recovery efforts. He simply said he wanted to see me every three months for the next year and would order a CT scan every three months.

He provided no insight into what we should do, so we developed our own plan—a ramp-up plan to improve my blood counts, stamina and strength. With as low a survival rate as esophageal cancer had, I thought there was a high probability the cancer would return or show up in my liver, kidney, lungs or bones. Our recovery plan focused on getting and keeping me as physically strong and healthy as possible should my cancer return and require another treatment round.

Find What Works for You

Decide to Live and you decide *not* to let cancer take over your life. How you decide to live with cancer is your choice, and the decision will return your personal power. Find what works for you.

Several things worked for me and the first was music. I assembled specific groups of songs by various artists who I felt depicted my point of view and attitude about cancer:

"It's a Great Day to be Alive" by Travis Tritt

"Center Field" by John Fogerty

"Shape I'm In" by the Arc Angels

"How Sweet It Is" by James Taylor

The song I heard in my head most often was "Center Field," specifically the verse, "Put me in coach, I'm ready to play today." I sang this song going into treatment, and these lyrics were the last words I remember saying to the surgeon when they administered the anesthesia to put me out. **Music worked for me.**

The second thing that worked for me was my attitude that I wasn't dying; I just had cancer. It sounded like a country-western song, but it worked for me.

The third and most important thing was my sense of humor. It helped me get through treatment when things were really rough.

Decide to Live and you establish a mind-set that makes a difference and provides the motivation and strength you need to get through treatment.

Section II: Developing a Course of Action

Final Notes

The messages in *One Tough Journey* are intended to help you and your caregiver through your cancer treatment journey. When I started my journey, who knew how it would end?

At the time of this writing, it's been more than three years since my diagnosis and more than two since I completed my last round of chemo. My last PET and CT scans confirmed I am cancer free—hooray for our side!—and the staff at the cancer center now calls Linda and me by our *first* names.

Recovery took longer than I expected. I still have major side effects that may never go away: The ends of my fingers and toes have no feeling, and I must be very careful to protect them from frost bite in colder weather. My body hair hasn't completely returned. I have major bald spots on my scalp, and my eyebrows have not grown back. My sense of taste hasn't returned, and I'm still lactose intolerant.

But my body weight has returned to normal, my energy level has returned slowly and I've regained much of my physical strength, though my stamina is still a little weak—maybe because I'm older. To facilitate recovery, I expanded my weight-lifting workout and added more protein to my diet. I still eat six meals a day, including lots of antioxidant-rich fruits and vegetables. Because esophageal cancer is fast acting, my infusion port is still in place just in case. I have it flushed every three months and also have a CT scan every three months.

I believe four factors contributed to my survival:

My physical strength — It helped me endure chemo, radiation, surgery and a second session of chemo and helped me stay healthy so treatment was never halted.

My wife and caregiver, Linda — She wouldn't take any crap from me, pushed me when I needed it and worked with me through the treatment and recovery process.

My oncologist, Dr. Greco, and his cancer treatment team — They aggressively treated my cancer at The Center for Cancer Care and Research in St. Louis, Missouri, and provided the highest level of medical care and service.

My personal motivation not to give up the fight — The abundant prayers of my family and friends inspired me and helped me believe I could win this fight.

My final coaching note again stresses the importance of maintaining and protecting your caregiver's health and well being. The cancer treatment journey is extremely stressful for caregivers and can take a heavy toll. Help your caregiver recognize their new responsibility, which gives them a new purpose, too. Even though caregivers don't go through treatment, accompanying those of us who do requires strength and good health—for caregivers and patients alike.

Use *One Tough Journey* to your advantage and build on it. Every cancer patient knows something another cancer patient can benefit from. Sharing your knowledge may someday help another cancer patient who is just beginning *one tough journey*.

Coach4Cancer™ was established to assist cancer patients and their caregivers through the treatment and recovery journey.

It seeks to provide information, encouragement and motivation to improve the ability of patients to endure treatment and defeat their cancer. For more information, visit the website:

www.coach4cancer.com

Section III:
Summary of Principles

*This section summarizes the Must Get Rights,
its principles and concepts, and includes charts,
forms and templates for your use during treatment.*

C4C — oach **4** ancer™

One Tough Journey

Now Begins the Toughest Battle of Your Life and for Your Life

Surviving cancer requires proactive participation. Your cancer team will play offense and do everything possible to help you beat the cancer. It's incumbent on you to play the best *defensive* game to help your body endure the treatment.

If you ever needed a cause to rally for, this is it. Today, more patients survive cancer than ever before, and you can be one of them. The challenge you face is to survive treatment, live through it and become stronger.

How to Fight the Battle

- Develop a survivor's attitude to challenge a formidable, relentless enemy
- Decide you are not sick — you just have cancer
- Learn to manage the fear factor and realize you do have choices
- Make every effort to stay healthy during treatment and recovery
- Ask questions; don't be afraid to challenge your oncologist and cancer treatment team
- Avoid feeling like a victim by becoming a knowledgeable patient
- Join the journey — proactively participate in your treatment
- Believe you can win this fight

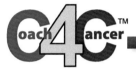

Must Get Rights

- Participate Proactively
- Be Knowledgeable
- Reduce the Fear Factor

Join the Journey

Feed the System

Decide to Live

- Eat Well for Strength
- Stay Active
- Develop Mental Fortitude

- Stay Engaged
- Buck up When Necessary
- Show Your Inner Strength

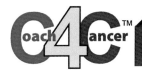

Must Get Rights

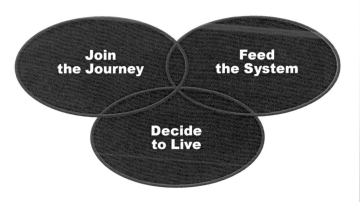

Challenge Your Cancer
Put it on Notice
You are in for the Fight

Join the Journey

Proactive Participation	Knowledgeable Patient
• Engage Your Oncologist and Cancer Treatment Team	• Research and Know Your Cancer Treatment and Its Side Effects
• Learn the Treatment Process	• Know Your Treatment and Test Alternatives
• Listen to Your Body	• Learn About Current Successes
• Prepare for Treatment	
• Dress for Comfort and Warmth	• Learn About Foods and Beverages Rich in Antioxidants
• Make Notes and Prepare Questions	• Recognize Your Temperament
	• Recognize the Toll on Your Caregiver

Find What Works for You

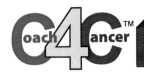

Must Get Rights

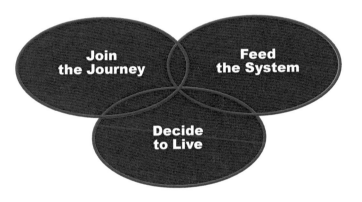

Join the Journey

Feed the System

Decide to Live

A Weak Soldier
Cannot Survive
a Long Physical Battle

Feed the System

Nutritional	Physical	Mental
• Eat Well for Treatment and Recovery	• Be Ready for Treatment	• Be Positive; Cancer Is not a Death Sentence
• Eat Four to Six Small Meals a Day	• Continue Your Normal Activities	• Dig Deep Into Your Inner Strength
• Eat More Protein	• Exercise and Play	
• Add Vitamins to Your Diet	• Sleep to Recover	• Embrace Your New Purpose
• Drink More Water	• Rest When Tired	
• Have an Alcoholic Beverage	• Work at Your Job	• Settle Your Emotions
	• Manage the Pain; It Will Pass	• Recognize Your Mortality
	• Document and Track Your Side Effects	• Stay Motivated
	• Nausea is Temporary	• Celebrate Small Triumphs
	• Hair Loss is Temporary	• Use Prayer for Strength
	• Stay Warm	• Plan Your Activities
	• Stay Healthy	

Find What Works for You

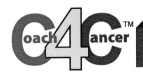

Cancer is Not a Final Destination – It is a Journey

Must Get Rights

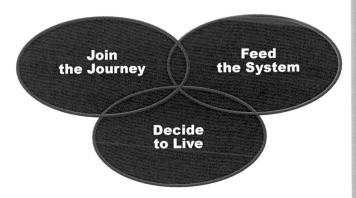

Challenge Your Cancer
Put it on Notice
You are in for the Fight

Decide to Live

Stay Engaged	Get an Attitude
• Buck Up	• Stay Connected with Your Social and Family Networks
• Believe You Can Win the Fight	• Challenge the Cancer
• Regain Your Personal Power	• Do New Things
• Continue with Your Life	• Choose Not to be a Victim
• Celebrate the Good Days and Push Through the Bad	• Don't Get Discouraged
	• Recover to Live
	• Call on Your Sense of Humor

Find What Works for You

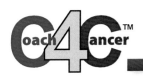

Cancer Diagnosis and Treatment Plan

Chart I

Page ___ of ___

Record your diagnosis, treatment plan and the names and phone numbers of your cancer treatment team.

Name: _____

Date: _____

Cancer Diagnosis

Type: _____

Stage: _____

Grade: _____

Primary Physician: _____ Office _____ **Other Contacts**

_____ Exchange _____ _____

Oncologist: _____ Office _____ _____

_____ Exchange _____ _____

Nurse Practitioner _____ _____

_____ Office _____ _____

Radiologist: _____ Office _____ _____

_____ Exchange _____ _____

Nurse Practitioner _____ _____

_____ Office _____ _____

Surgeon: _____ Office _____ _____

_____ Exchange _____ _____

Nurse Practitioner _____ _____

_____ Office _____ _____

Name of Treatment Protocol: _____

Name of Clinical Trial: _____

Summary of Prescribed Treatment Plan

Chemotherapy

_____

_____

_____

_____

_____

_____

_____

Radiation

_____

_____

_____

_____

_____

_____

_____

Surgery

_____

_____

_____

_____

_____

_____

_____

© 2008 by LCJ Enterprises, LLC. All rights reserved.

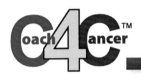

Treatment Schedule

Chart II

Name: _____

Record your treatment, test and doctor appointments.

Month: _____

Sun	Mon	Tues	Wed	Thurs	Fri	Sat

Month: _____

Sun	Mon	Tues	Wed	Thurs	Fri	Sat

Month: _____

Sun	Mon	Tues	Wed	Thurs	Fri	Sat

Month: _____

Sun	Mon	Tues	Wed	Thurs	Fri	Sat

© 2008 by LCJ Enterprises, LLC. All rights reserved.

Chart III

Summary Of Current Medications

Name: _____

Medication Name	Dosage	Medication Purpose	Application Frequency	Prescribing Physician

List all prescription medications, over-the-counter medications, vitamins, herbal supplements, meal substitute drinks and protein drinks.

© 2008 by LCJ Enterprises, LLC. All rights reserved.08

Ask questions to become a proactive participant in your treatment.

- How long have you treated cancer patients?
- Why should you be on my treatment team?
- Have you treated this type of cancer before?
- What success have you had with it?
- What is the survival rate?
- What treatment do you prescribe?
- Where was it developed and used?
- Why are you prescribing it?
- What are the past results?
- How long does treatment last?
- What are my treatment options and alternatives?
- What are the success rates of the treatment options and alternatives?
- What's the best treatment facility for this cancer?
- Should I get a second opinion?
- Who is the lead physician for my treatment?

- Does my health insurance limit coverage for treatment?
- Where do I learn more about my cancer and prescribed treatment?
- Why do I need these tests?
- What will the test results tell you?
- What do you see on the x-ray?
- What do the blood analysis numbers tell you?
- What should I look for?
- Will treatment damage other parts of my body?
- Can it damage other organs?
- What can I do to protect myself?
- Where would infection show up?
- How do I combat the side effects?
- How long will the side effects last?
- How will I know if the cancer has returned?
- Are we winning yet?

© 2008 by LCJ Enterprises, LLC. All rights reserved.

Chart V

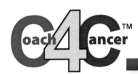

Journal of Physical Health

Date and record changes in your physical health, such as numbness, bleeding, weakness or other changes you experience, including changes in their intensity and frequency.

Date	Description of Physical Changes	Intensity Low to High 1 2 3 4 5	Frequency

© 2008 by LCJ Enterprises, LLC. All rights reserved.

Chart VI

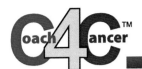 **Journal of Notes and Questions**

Put an X under the topics your treatment notes and questions cover.

Resolved ✔	Date: _____	Allergic Reaction	Bleeding	Caregiver	Emotions	Fatigue	Fear	Fever	Infections	Inoculations	Medication	Medical Expenses	Pain	Physical Health	Senses	Schedules	Side Effects	Sores	Specialists	Strength	Treatment	Other
	Note 1 ---- Question																					
	Note 2 ---- Question																					
	Note 3 ---- Question																					
	Note 4 ---- Question																					
	Note 5 ---- Question																					
	Note 6 ---- Question																					
	Note 7 ---- Question																					
	Note 8 ---- Question																					
	Note 9 ---- Question																					
	Note 10 ---- Question																					

© 2008 by LCJ Enterprises, LLC. All rights reserved.

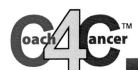

Chart VII

Treatment Preparation Action Plan

Use this chart to prepare for treatment and to plan how you'll use the time.

Treatment Round _____ **Treatment Dates** _____ **Treatment Duration** _____

Pre-Treatment Preparation

Exercise	_____	Vitamins	_____
	_____		_____
	_____		_____
Meal	_____	Bodily	_____
	_____	Functions	_____
Clothing	_____	Other	_____
	_____		_____
	_____		_____
Medication	_____		_____
	_____		_____

Pack for Treatment

Reading Material	_____	Cell Phone	_____
Newspapers	_____	Computer	_____
Magazines	_____	CD Player	_____
Books	_____	Earphones	_____
Other	_____	Portable TV	_____
Food & Snacks	_____	Radio	_____
		Other	_____
Beverages	_____		
Hobby Supplies	_____		_____
Writing Supplies	_____		_____

Activities During Treatment

- _____
- _____
- _____
- _____
- _____
- _____
- _____

- _____
- _____
- _____
- _____
- _____
- _____
- _____

© 2008 by LCJ Enterprises, LLC. All rights reserved.

Chart VIII
Page 1 of 2

C4C™ Medical Appointment Agenda

Coach4Cancer

Use this chart to prepare for your oncology appointments.

Appointment Date: _____ **Time:** _____ **Physician:** _____

Purpose: _____ **Pre-appt. Time** _____

SUMMARY OF PHYSICAL HEALTH Rank Side Effects: Low (1 2 3 4 5) High

Allergic Reaction _____	Diarrhea _____	Indigestion _____	Pain _____	Strength _____
Appetite Loss _____	Dizziness _____	Infection _____	Physical Health _____	Sweating _____
Bleeding _____	Dry Mouth _____	Inoculations _____	Rash _____	Swelling _____
Bruising _____	Dry Skin/Itching _____	Insomnia _____	Sensory Changes _____	Tearing _____
Burning Sensation _____	Emotions _____	Intestinal Gas _____	Shortness of Breath _____	Throat Irritation _____
Caregiver's Health _____	Energy Level _____	Joint/Muscle Pain _____	Side Effects _____	Tingling _____
Chemo Brain _____	Fatigue _____	Medical Expenses _____	Sense of Smell _____	Transportation _____
Chills _____	Fear _____	Medications _____	Sense of Taste _____	Treatment _____
Concentration _____	Fever _____	Mouth Sores _____	Sores _____	Vomiting _____
Constipation _____	Fluid Retention _____	Nail Changes _____	Stiffness _____	Wheezing _____
Coughing _____	Hair Loss _____	Nausea _____	Stomach Cramps _____	Other _____
	Headache _____	Numbness _____		

Questions

1. _____
2. _____
3. _____
4. _____
5. _____
6. _____
7. _____

Answers

1. _____
2. _____
3. _____
4. _____
5. _____
6. _____
7. _____

© 2008 by LCJ Enterprises, LLC. All rights reserved.

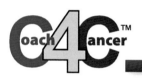

Use this chart to record the results of every medical appointment.

Physician's Overall Medical Evaluation

Progress Report

Prescribed Next Steps

© 2008 by LCJ Enterprises, LLC. All rights reserved.

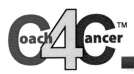

Journal of Treatment Side Effects

Chart IX

Page _____ of _____

Rank each side effect with the appropriate level of intensity. Summarize how you feel and write down any questions.

Rank Side Effects: Low (1 2 3 4 5) High

Date	Allergic Reaction	Appetite Loss	Bleeding	Bruising	Burning Sensation	Chemo Brain	Chills	Concentration	Constipation	Cough	Diarrhea	Dizziness	Dry Mouth	Dry Skin/Itching	Energy Level	Fatigue	Fever	Fluid Retention	Hair Loss	Headache	Indigestion	Infection	Insomnia	Intestinal Gas	Joint Pain	Mouth Sores	Muscle Pain	Nail Changes	Nausea	Rash	Shortness of Breath	Sense of Smell	Sense of Taste	Sores	Stiffness	Stomach Cramps	Strength	Sweating	Swelling	Tearing	Throat Irritation	Tingling & Numbness	Vomiting	Wheezing	Other Side Effects

Overall Health Summary

- _____
- _____
- _____
- _____
- _____
- _____
- _____

Questions to Ask

1. _____
2. _____
3. _____
4. _____
5. _____
6. _____
7. _____

© 2008 by LCJ Enterprises, LLC. All rights reserved.

Chart X

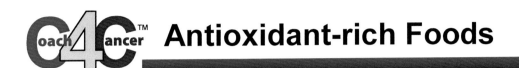 **Antioxidant-rich Foods**

Berry Fruits
Blackberries
Blueberries
Strawberries
Raspberries
Cherries
Cranberries

Citrus Fruits
Oranges
Kiwis
Pineapple
Red Grapefruit
Lemons
Limes

Other Fruits
Apples & Apricots
Mangos & Peaches
Prunes & Plums
Watermelon & Cantaloupe
Red Grapes
Tomatoes
Raisins

Beverages
Green & White Tea
Coffee
V-8 Juice
Dark Beer
Red Wine
Pomegranate Juice

Vegetables
Broccoli & Cauliflower
Brussels Sprouts
Spinach
Green & Red Peppers
Sweet Potatoes
Artichoke (Cooked)
Cabbage
Squash
Carrots
Pumpkin

Proteins
Fish & Shellfish
Chicken
Lean Red Meats
Calf's Liver
Beans
Eggs
Pecans & Walnuts
Almonds
Peanuts
Soy Nuts
Sunflower Seeds

Grains & Cereals
Whole Grains
Oatmeal
Barley
Rice
Rye
Flaxseed
Rice Cereal

Spices
Cinnamon
Oregano
Parsley
Paprika
Black Pepper
Honey

Chart XI

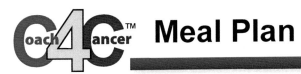 **Meal Plan**

	Breakfast	Morning Snack	Lunch	Afternoon Snack	Dinner	Bedtime Snack	Calories
Sunday Menu							
Total Calories							
Monday Menu							
Total Calories							
Tuesday Menu							
Total Calories							
Wednesday Menu							
Total Calories							
Thursday Menu							
Total Calories							
Friday Menu							
Total Calories							
Saturday Menu							
Total Calories							

Chart XII
Page 1 of 2

Recovery Plan and Journal

Coach 4 Cancer™

Record your diagnosis, treatment plan and the names and phone numbers of your cancer treatment team.

Name: _____

Date: _____

Treatment Completion Date: _____

Cancer Diagnosis Date: _____

Type: _____

Stage: _____

Grade: _____

	Office		Other Contacts
Primary Physician:	Office _____		_____
	Exchange _____		_____
Oncologist:	Office _____		_____
	Exchange _____		_____
Nurse Practitioner _____			_____
	Office _____		_____
Radiologist:	Office _____		_____
	Exchange _____		_____
Nurse Practitioner _____			_____
	Office _____		_____
Surgeon:	Office _____		_____
	Exchange _____		_____
Nurse Practitioner _____			_____
	Office _____		_____

Summary of Prescribed Treatment Plan

Chemotherapy Summary: _____

_____

_____

Radiation Summary: _____

_____

Other Treatment Summary: _____

Surgery Summary: _____

_____

_____

Summary of Complications and Major Side Effects: _____

_____

© 2008 by LCJ Enterprises, LLC. All rights reserved.

Chart XII
Page 2 of 2

Recovery Plan and Journal

Recovery Follow-up Plan

	3 months	6 months	9 months	12 months
Observation & Surveillance for Recurrence				
Long-term & Late Effects Monitoring				
Secondary Cancer Surveillance				
Port Flush				
Additional Recommendations				

Recovery Journal

Nutrition Meals Calories Vitamins Protein Other				
Physical Requirements Exercise Workouts Other Activities				
Sleep				
Work				
Relaxation Activities				

© 2008 by LCJ Enterprises, LLC. All rights reserved.

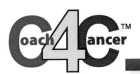

Recovery Schedule

Chart XIII

Name: _____

Record your appointment schedule for follow-up tests, scans and reviews with your treatment team.

Month: _____

Sun	Mon	Tues	Wed	Thurs	Fri	Sat

Month: _____

Sun	Mon	Tues	Wed	Thurs	Fri	Sat

Month: _____

Sun	Mon	Tues	Wed	Thurs	Fri	Sat

Month: _____

Sun	Mon	Tues	Wed	Thurs	Fri	Sat

© 2008 by LCJ Enterprises, LLC. All rights reserved.

Chart XIV

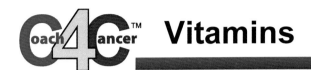 **Vitamins**

You may want to include the following vitamins and supplements during treatment and recovery. Be sure to discuss your supplement choices with your doctor to avoid conflicts with your treatment regimen.

- Multivitamin (be sure it includes iron to help build red-blood cells)

- Vitamin A (people with cancer require higher-than-normal amounts of this antioxidant)

- Vitamin B-complex (aids liver function, helps build red blood cells and improves circulation)

- Vitamin E (a powerful antioxidant and cancer-fighting agent)

- Vitamin C (powerful cancer-fighting agent that promotes the production of interferon in the body)

- CoQ10 (improves cellular oxygenation).

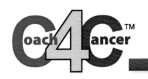

Resources

Chart XV

The following resources may help increase your knowledge and understanding of cancer, cancer treatments, statistics, trials, tests and other relevant information, including links to organizations that address specific cancers and treatments.

National Cancer Institute
Bethesda, MA
800-422-6237
cancer.gov

American Cancer Society
Atlanta, GA (home office)
800-227-2345
cancer.org

LIVESTRONG
Lance Armstrong Foundation
Austin, TX 75219
866-235-7205
livestrong.org

Nature's Best
195 Engineers Road
Hauppauge, NY 11788
naturesbest.com

The Center for Cancer Care and Research
12855 North Forty Dr. Suite 200
St. Louis, MO 63141
314-628-1210
tcccr.com

The Wellness Community of Greater St. Louis
1058 Old Des Peres Rd.
St. Louis, MO 63131
314-238-2000
wellnesscommunitystl.org

CURE: Cancer Updates, Research & Education
(a quarterly publication of CURE Media Group, LP)
3102 Oak Lawn Avenue, Suite 610
Dallas, TX 75219
800-210-CURE (2873); 214-367-3500
curetoday.com and **curemediagroup.com**

Comprehensive resource of cancer websites
cancer.com